CBD FOR PETS

A Guide to Pet Wellness with CBD

HOW PETS ARE FINDING RELIEF FROM ANXIETY, INFLAMMATION & AGING PAINS

Dean Killingbeck

CBD for Pets: A Guide to Pet Wellness with CBD

Copyright © 2020 by Dean Killingbeck

Dedication

This book is dedicated to all the pet shelter volunteers who dedicate thousands of hours of their lives every year helping pets. This world is a better and more compassionate place because of you.

Thank you.

Table of Contents

Part I: The Science of CBD

Part II: Pet Parent Tell Their CBD Stories

Part III: Resources

Introduction
by Dean Killingbeck

CBD is changing the wellness landscape for pets. Whether you have a dog or cat; aging or still young; recovering from health problems or just suffering from anxiety....

You owe it to your pet to understand how hemp and CBD, made by nature can help you pet live healthier and longer.

I wrote this book because I felt there is a huge need for pet parents to understand how CBD and hemp can help their pets. CBD is not a cure-all nor can it fix every health problem that a pet might encounter during their lives with us but its wellness benefits are many and overall I believe it can help both cats and dogs in many different ways.

Dean

The author, seen here at harvest of 2019 hemp crop in Michigan

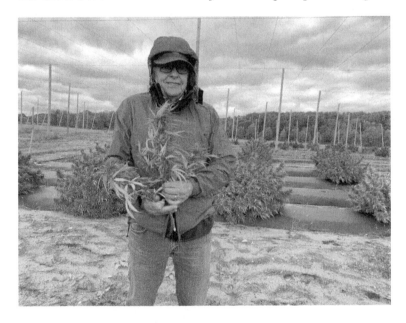

Chapter One
What is CBD?

CBD stands for cannabidiol, which is a compound extracted from the hemp plant. It's one of the 113 cannabinoids, which are naturally occurring unique compounds found in the cannabis & hemp family of plants.

Hemp has been cultivated for its medicinal, psychoactive, and physical properties for thousands of years. The earliest recorded medicinal uses of the plant date as far back as 1400-2,000 BC.

What can CBD do for your pets?

The first time CBD broke into national news was it being successfully used to stop seizures in children suffering from rare form of epilepsy. Since then CBD has exploded in popularity globally as an all-natural plant based ingredient for humans and pets.

Millions of people are using CBD oil every day to reduce anxiety, sleep better and more deeply and decrease pain due to inflammation in your body. Think of CBD as the ultimate guide built by nature over millions of years that will bring your body and mental states back in harmony and balance.

For pets especially dogs and cats, growing number of pets parents are successfully using CBD to help their pets with decreasing anxiety (from loud sounds, fireworks, separation fears from their pet parent, travel, going to vet); reduce inflammation in skin & coat; , regain appetite lost to chemo or aging; and help with aging discomforts such as aging joint and muscle pains.

CBD for pet products come in many forms: tinctures, treats, sprays, capsules and even soothing balms for inflamed paws.

Does CBD come from marijuana?

It's true that hemp and marijuana both come from the same plant family, Cannabis sativa L. but they have some significant differences.

The hemp family of plants is bred by farmers to have high concentrations of CBD, but contains only traces amount of THC, less than 0.3% as required by US Government Farm Bill 2018.

Have less than 0.3% THC is the only way CBD products could be sold freely via stores and online, shipped through States and even exported without the massive restrictions that the marijuana industry faces in selling their marijuana products which can be purchased from local marijuana dispensaries and no inter-State sales are allowed.

On the other hand marijuana plants are bred to be high in THC and has lower levels of CBD. It's much like lemons and oranges. They are both belong to citrus family and so they have some familiarity but they are two different plants with 2 different flavors.

Can my pets get high with CBD?

No. CBD is not marijuana and your pet can't get high from taking CBD hemp oil. It's extracted from hemp, which contains less than 0.3% THC so your pet's body cannot physically consume the amount needed to ever get high.

Remember the last time you ate a lot of fried food and felt sleepy as your body was trying to digest all the oil you took. Almost all CBD products are CBD mixed up with some type of carrier oil: MCT, hemp or olive oil. If you give your pet too much CBD oil, they will probably fall asleep as their body is trying to digest all that oil but not get high.

So how come my bottle of CBD smell like cannabis?

Hemp and Marijuana both come from the same plant family, Cannabis sativa L. and they both contain terpenes. Terpenes are what you smell. Secreted in the same glands that produce cannabinoids like THC and CBD, terpenes are aromatic oils that color cannabis varieties (hemp included) and even in tiny amounts, terpenes work extremely well with cannabinoids to heal the body, and are a contributing factor to the *"entourage effect"* in our CBD which is all the compounds found naturally in the hemp plant working together to bring maximum wellness to a pet or human body.

Sure you can chemically remove THC from the oils extracted from the hemp or even vaporize every other compound and bottle just CBD in a bottle and make it smell like orange juice but when you do that, you are leaving so much more wellness benefits out of your CBD product.

The *entourage effect* is the main difference between using a full spectrum CBD product (all the compounds including the 0.3% THC coming naturally from the hemp plant) vs using Isolate based products which is just CBD powder, chemically extracted from the hemp plant by itself and then mixed with some kind of oil.

Will a full spectrum CBD with 0.3% THC show up on a drug test for humans?

Although pets don't have to worry about drug testing, pet parents do. Much like the consumption of poppy seeds may lead to a positive drug test for opioids, the consumption of certain hemp products may lead to a positive drug test for tetrahydrocannabinol (THC).

THC is inherently present in trace amounts in hemp plants. The legal limit of THC in hemp is no more than 0.3%.

For pet parents who are subjected to regular drug testing (truck drivers, law enforcement, public safety for example) we strongly suggest consulting your health care provider before consuming any hemp products because individual biochemistry, the potential for the conversion of cannabinoids, and the possibility of trace, but legal, amounts of THC inherent in hemp products are all factors to consider before using any kind of product made from the hemp plant.

Expect drug testing to evolve in the next few years to understand the difference between getting high and taking CBD for pain. Till then, check with your health care provider of your employers before taking any CBD products for yourself.

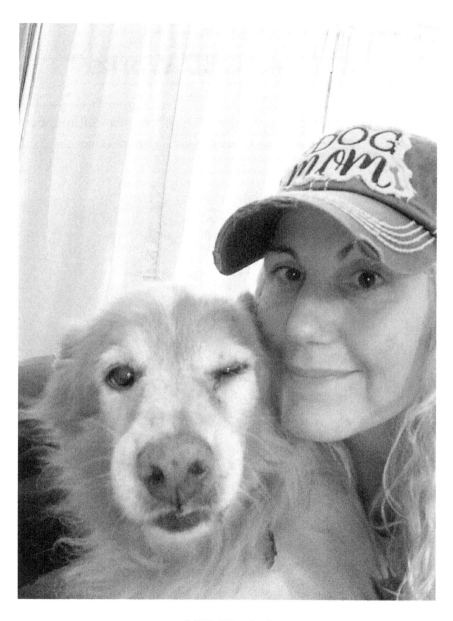

CBD Works!

"I just wanted to relay our experience. I received the oil on the day that my old guy couldn't even stand up on his own. And that was after a couple of days of limping. I gave him a dose, and 45 min. later, he stood up on his own. After 3 days of 2X a day dosing, he was 100 times better!!!" – Mary Harp, Michigan

Chapter Two
How Does CBD Works?

How can one molecule do that all that? Reduce inflammation. Reduce anxiety. Bring comfort to aging pets. It almost sounds too good to be true.

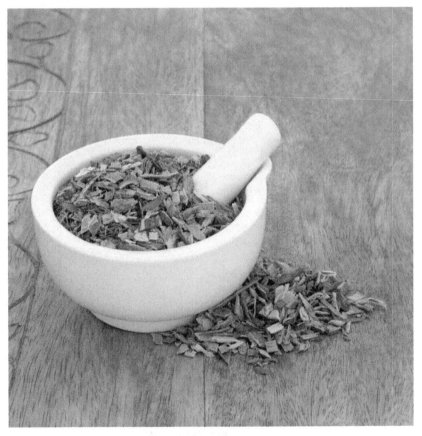

Willow Bark to Aspirin

There is another plant based medicine, that was used for thousands of years before scientists were able to understand it and put it in a bottle for millions to use. Willow bark AKA Aspirin.

The use of willow bark for bringing pain relief dates as far as to the time of Hippocrates (400 BC) when healers advised people to chew on the bark to reduce fever and inflammation.

Willow bark has been used throughout the centuries in China and Europe, and continues to be used today for the treatment of pain, headaches and inflammatory conditions in many cultures. The bark of white willow contains Salicin and in the 1800s, Salicin was used to develop aspirin, another medicine that was viewed with suspicion from the medical community at that time and its healing properties questioned.

Similarly, hundreds of cultures from India to Latin America have been using the cannabis family of plants that also includes hemp for wellness benefits for thousands of years.

The science and research into CBD and THC have been non-existent because hemp was lumped with marijuana and got effectively banned from research institutions in USA. It is only recently that scientists have began to unravel what nature has gifted us with.

What is Homeostasis?

What does your body do every day, every night, every second? It seeks balance. When you become too hot, your body produces sweat to cool you down. When your blood sugar becomes elevated after a meal, your body secretes insulin to lower it. And when you become dehydrated, your body sends your brain thirst signals so you drink water. These are all examples of homeostasis.

The therapeutic magic of CBD and, in some cases, THC — and maybe some of the more than 100 other cannabinoids in cannabis — may come from the ways that, by tweaking the endocannabinoid system, they push the body away from disease toward the unruffled state scientists call homeostasis.

Homeostasis is the mammal's body regulation of conditions that exist naturally in the body every day, every moment: body temperature, blood sugar level, water content are just some examples of Homeostasis in action. Our bodies, pets included are always moving toward that unruffled state balance.

So how does our and our pets bodies achieve that balance? We maintain homeostasis by using negative feedback mechanisms. This means that everything in our bodies is monitored carefully so that, when something is out of balance (need water for example) our bodies alert us and ask us to correct that condition. This is where the endocannabinoid system comes in.

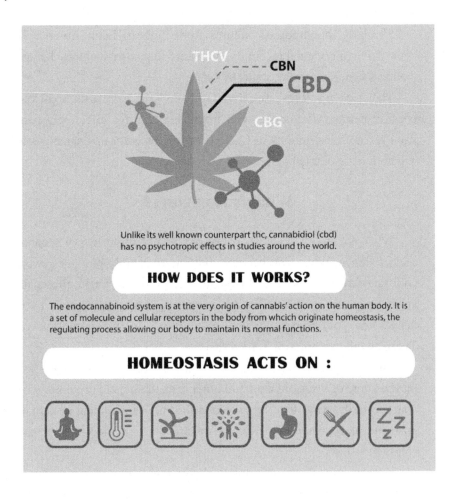

Unlike its well known counterpart thc, cannabidiol (cbd) has no psychotropic effects in studies around the world.

HOW DOES IT WORKS?

The endocannabinoid system is at the very origin of cannabis' action on the human body. It is a set of molecule and cellular receptors in the body from whcich originate homeostasis, the regulating process allowing our body to maintain its normal functions.

HOMEOSTASIS ACTS ON :

What is the Endocannabinoid System?

The endocannabinoid system is a network of endocannabinoids and cannabinoid receptors that exist throughout our bodies. It is thought to exist in pretty much all animals on earth, and it is absolutely crucial to our survival.

The cannabinoid receptors exist on the surface of cells and "listen" to what's going on in the body. They communicate this information about

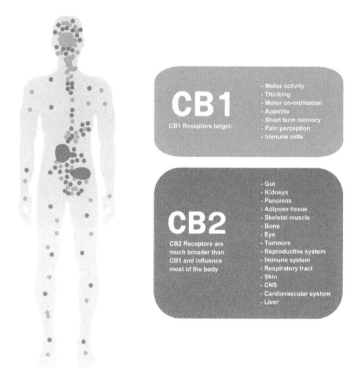

our bodies' status and changing circumstances to the inside of the cell, allowing for the appropriate measures to be taken.

So far scientists have identified two types of primary cannabinoid receptors, called the CB1 and CB2 receptors. Although both types of receptors can be found all throughout the body, CB1 receptors are more highly concentrated in the brain and central nervous system, whereas

CB2 receptors can be found more abundantly in the immune system, organs, and tissues.

Like a hemp plant, a mammals body (pets and people) also produces its own cannabinoids, which are referred to as endocannabinoids. These molecules are created whenever we need them, usually in response to some change in the body.

Chapter Three

How can CBD help pets?

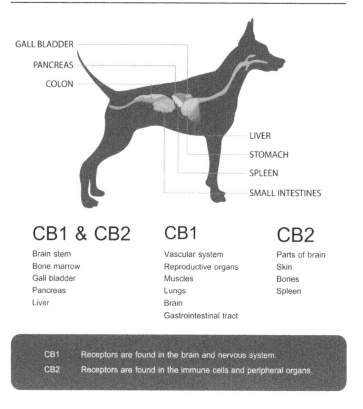

YOU DOGS CANNABINOID RECEPTRS

CB1 & CB2	CB1	CB2
Brain stem	Vascular system	Parts of brain
Bone marrow	Reproductive organs	Skin
Gall bladder	Muscles	Bones
Pancreas	Lungs	Spleen
Liver	Brain	
	Gastrointestinal tract	

CB1   Receptors are found in the brain and nervous system.
CB2   Receptors are found in the immune cells and peripheral organs.

How does CBD interact with the endocannabinoid system in a pets or our body?

When marijuana is consumed, the THC can bind directly with cannabinoid receptors, in the same way as our endocannabinoids do.

THC seems to have a preference for our CB1 receptors, found in the brain, which is why THC can cause psychoactive, intoxicating effects and make its users high and hungry.

Cannabidiol or CBD acts differently from THC. Instead of binding directly with our cannabinoid receptors, CBD binds with an indirect influence on the ECS to produce more endocannabinoids naturally, which in turn leads to a better functioning of the endocannabinoid system and a healthier body for our pets and us.

YOUR CATS CANNABINOID RECEPTORS

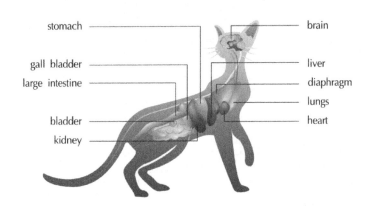

stomach — brain
gall bladder — liver
large intestine — diaphragm
— lungs
bladder — heart
kidney

CB1 & CB2	CB1	CB2
Gall Bladder	Brain	Bones
Brain Stem	Gastrointestinal tract	Brain
Bone Marrow	Lungs	Spleen
Liver	Muscles	Skin
Pancreas	Reproductive Organs	
	Vascular System	

CB1   Receptors are predominantly found in the brain and nervous system.
CB2   Receptors are predominantly found in the immune cells and peripheral organs.

Less Anxiety

Anxiety in pets comes in many forms. Separation from their pet parent, fear of going to veterinarian, fear of strangers and from loud noises especially thunder and fireworks all different kinds of anxiety that affect both cats and dogs. Anxiety from strangers is even manifested more in pets that are rescued from abusive environments and then adopted.

CBD has shown to produce a calming effect in pets from all the above forms of anxiety. It does not make a pet 'high' nor does it induces an early nap time for them. Instead it brings a sense of balance and calmness to pets. It even helps pets in minimizing aggression towards other animals and people mostly caused by some type of anxiety.

Read Chapter Five about pet parent stories about successfully trying CBD for different types of anxiety.

Less Aging Discomforts

Just like their pet parents, pets also experience discomfort in their muscles, joints and bones as they age. These aches convince pets that it might be better not to move at all and just lie all day on a couch or on their favorite corner. Not only this lack of mobility creates unhealthy weight gains in pets but also creates less flexibility in muscles and joints. Not moving around, not being active is not the solution to any kind of aches and pains but actually creates even more mobility pains with them.

CBD has powerful anti-inflammatory qualities that help to reduce swelling in the joints and muscles and can help get them moving around again. One of the most common and delightful comment is a pet parent saying: "Hey my 13 year old dog thinks he is a puppy again."

Read Chapter 13 about pet parent stories about some incredible stories on how CBD has bought relief from again discomforts to their pets.

Better Appetite

Many pets can experience a loss of appetite with aging. Pets undergoing chemotherapy for cancer treatments experience major drops in appetite and increased nausea which in turns creates nutrition and weight loss problems. The medical marijuana legalization movement started with chemotherapy patients in California discovering that marijuana was the only solution to their consistent nausea and loss of appetite. Full spectrum CBD products with .3% THC can help pets to boost their appetite, reduce nausea, and help with other digestive issues as well.

Read Chapter Ten about CBD helping pets with better digestion and appetite.

Less Inflammation

The sight of a dog or cat scratching their skin or coat into a frenzy will hurt your heart even if you are not a pet parent. Severe inflammation of skin & coat is a problem that hurts pets of all breeds, sizes and age. CBD is a natural super anti-inflammation agent and interacts with receptors inside a pet's body (just like with a human's body) to boost the immune system and bring immediate relief from severe itching and scratching to both dogs and cats.

Read Chapter Seven about CBD helping pets with severe skin & coat inflammation.

Chapter Four

All CBD Is Not Created Equal... The 5 Things You Need To Know About CBD

Many suppliers would have you believe that all CBD products are the same or created equally. This is ABSOULTELY NOT TRUE!! Just like other products that you purchase, some are of higher quality than others. So, to wade through the hype you must know these 5 things.

1. Is the CBD 3rd Party Tested?

Is the company having a 3rd party test their products to make sure that the CBD they're claiming is what is actually in the bottle. You must read their Certificate of Analysis otherwise known as COA to find out if their claims are true.

Example: I recently was working with a Chiropractor that was looking at switching to our products. After going online and seeing the company's COA's here's what I found: their 250 mg of CBD had 825 mg of CBD, their 750mg had 825mg of CBD and, their 1500mg had 825 mg of CBD.

All they did was change the label on their products. So, as a consumer if you bought the 250mg you were overdosing and if you bought the 1500mg you were under dosing. We are now enclosing our COA called "What's In Your Bottle" with every purchase to make sure that you as a consumer know exactly what you're getting.

2. Is the CBD Full Spectrum?

There are 3 major types of CBD in the market:

1. Isolate
2. Full spectrum
3. Broad Spectrum.

It truly makes a difference on which one you're using. Let me explain why: Isolates are products that are made by using a highly refined process leaving only pure CBD isolate in the form of a white power with which all the beneficial cannabinoids, terpenes, vitamins and omega oils have been removed except CBD.

Generally, these products contain 99+% pure CBD and do not have detectable levels of THC based on lab testing. Unlike full spectrum products, isolates do not produce benefits from the "entourage effect."

So, what is the entourage effect? This phenomenon, called the entourage effect, results when the many components within the cannabis plant interact with the human body to produce a stronger influence than any one of those components alone – it's a synergistic effect.

To understand the concept, think of it in terms of human interactions. We all have talents and abilities that are different than others. When partnerships are formed between two people, and abilities are combined, achievements can be made that were otherwise unimaginable.

When we combine multiple compounds in their natural state, we don't end up with the sum of each part; instead, we get a multiplying effect. All these different compounds can amplify each other's chemistry, making the overall plant more effective in addressing unwanted symptoms.

As it turns out, cannabis contains more active compounds than just THC. Over 110 cannabinoids, terpenes, and omega fats have been found to work in conjunction with THC to produce the relief that is often reported by cannabis users. NOTE: to be considered as Hemp not marijuana all CBD must have .03% THC or less which will never make you high, that's one of the reasons its legal in all 50 states and can be shipped to every state. Hemp, which contains the inverse ratio (more CBD than THC) can relieve symptoms without the psychoactive effect of marijuana. It won't get you high!

Full Spectrum CBD is processed by a CO_2 extraction method using high pressure and very low heat which results in a very clean product (without any residue of solvents) and, leaves all the 110 cannabinoids, terpene, vitamins, omega 3 and omega 6 in the CBD.

Yes, it does have a trace amount of THC... less than .03% but, this is a good thing because a recent study done at the Murphy Pain Center concluded recently that Full Spectrum CBD works best for pain relief and creates the entourage effect that is needed for full benefits. Full Spectrum is what we use in our products.

Broad Spectrum: This is again another highly processed product taking out all or most of the THC that nature gives us to heal our pet's bodies, "Why Fool With Nature?".

3. Make Sure Hemp is Grown in the USA

Lots of European brands get their CBD from China and Russia. Many cheap products sold in the USA are using these countries as their source of CBD. Why? You may ask... because its cheap! That's why gas stations, video stores, smoke shops, vape shops and others can advertise cheap product and, remember that the 3rd party testing I mentioned above, there isn't any.

Do we as pet parents want to give our best friends heavy metals, pesticides, herbicides, molds and other contaminants when we are trying to heal them or ourselves? "I really don't think so." NOTE: Hemp is considered a remediate plant and one researcher from Phytotech, Slavik Dushenkova, remarked that "hemp is proving to be one of the best phytoremediation - technologies that use living plants to clean up soil, air, and water contaminated with hazardous materials.

Phytotech is part of a group of research companies that are testing industrial hemp in an attempt to clean up the radioactive soil that surrounds Chernobyl. For the past decade, industrial hemp has been growing around the abandoned Chernobyl nuclear power plant in Pripyat, Ukraine, and has been helping to reduce soil toxicity. Is this where those cheap CBD companies are buying their hemp from? No one knows because no COAs are available.

4. Organically Grown and Free of Additives & Artificial Flavors

We all know that organically grown products are the best especially since we know that hemp is considered one of the best phytoremediation (plants that clean the soil). So, if its not organically grown and being sprayed with pesticides, herbicides and for mold, those chemicals are going into the ground and consequently into the plant.

This is another reason for 3rd party testing. Some put additives such as olive oil, coconut oil, grape seed oil, artificial coloring, or flavors into their oil. Example: Here's the additives in one such supplier - Purified Water, Vegetable Glycerin, Pollock Oil, Sunflower Lecithin, Xanthan Gum, Acacia Gum, Potassium Sorbate.

Why? This is strictly a marketing ploy attempting to say they have a better product by adding stuff into their CBD. We prefer to use organically grown hemp from Kentucky with all-natural hemp oil and CBD with no additives or colorings.

5. Read and Understand the Label

Wow, this is no easy task but its one that you really need to master because the label must list the ingredients of "What's In Your Bottle". In fact, many suppliers have NO CBD present or a minimum amount. Example: a well-known company has on its bottles "Hemp Oil 330" in big bold letters. At first look you would assume it has 330mg of CBD in it. Well, it actuality has only 100mg in the bottle. In order to discover what's in it you must look at the small print at the very bottom of the bottle. Illegal, no... mis-leading, yes! Which is why you must look at what's really in the bottle.

The amount of CBD in the bottle determines the dosage that's needed to solve you pets health problems so it's critical that you know. In fact, a 100mg CBD bottle with 3mg per full dropper used on a 60-100 pound dog with arthritis would require using 4 full droppers per day to achieve minimum results to alleviate the pain plus, the bottle would only last 7 days and that's at the minimum dosage.

Learn more about how to build the right dosage for your pet in the Resources section at the end of this book.

Example of Lab Report of CBD Oil Product

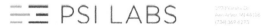

-- 500mg Tincture

Sample ID: 1904PSI0005.04180	Metrc ID:	Produced:	Pets Strong
Strain: - 500mg Tincture	-	Collected:	Lic. #
Matrix: Ingestible	Batch ID:	Completed: 04/03/2019	4341 Marwood Drive
Type: Other	PST03-01	Sample Size - : Batch -	Howell, MI 48855

Cannabinoids

<LOQ   **562.78**

Δ9-THC (mg/unit)   CBD (mg/unit)

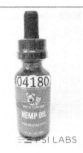

Testing Method: HPLC-DAD / SOP - PSIMTDA02
Date Tested: 04/03/2019
1 Unit = 1 fl oz, 27.8g

Analyte	LOQ	Mass	Mass
	mg/unit	mg/unit	mg/g
THCa	6.55	ND	ND
Δ9-THC	6.55	ND	ND
Δ8-THC	6.55	ND	ND
CBDa	6.55	ND	ND
CBD	6.55	562.78	20.24
CBN	6.55	ND	ND
Total		562.78	20.24

Chapter Five

Pet Anxiety and CBD Pet Parent Stories

A Rescue Pup Dealing With Terrible Anxiety

"Chesney is a three-year-old Great Pyrenees mix who I adopted from a shelter. Her skin was so infected and irritated, they actually believed she was a boy. Her whole body was just so inflamed and swollen. She was very sick. I set her up on a good food to start nursing her back to health, but early on, a trainer told me Chesney had really bad anxiety, and that it could be at the root of her symptoms."

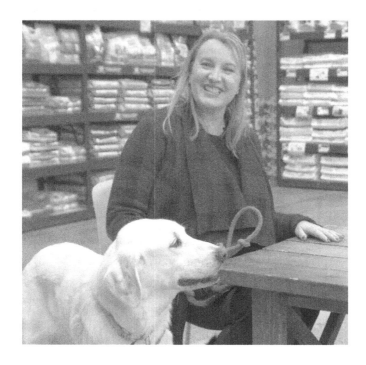

"We consulted a pet behaviorist at Michigan State who pointed out that there are eight major causes of anxiety, and Chesney had experienced all eight during her early life. For example, her mother wasn't able to produce the proper prenatal sustenance for her, Chesney had parvo as a puppy, and was separated way too early from her mother. It was clear: the anxiety that resulted from Chesney's early life of neglect is what was causing her body to be in constant malfunction and distress.

Our first solution was to try vet-prescribed Paxil, which helped a lot, but I also read about the benefits of CBD, and was excited to try it. I bought some CBD treats, and none of my dogs would eat them. They weren't cheap, and I was disappointed.

We then tried Xanax--also prescribed by the vet--but it had the opposite effect on her, which I guess is fairly common. It was literally like having a bucking rhinoceros in our living room. It was pretty sad. Daycare was almost impossible because she became really reactive. A dog attacked her and that changed her personality and increased her anxiety.

At that point, a pet nutritionist encouraged me to try CBD again, but this time in oil form. So I did, and it's heaven-sent! Great Pyrenees are pretty sensitive to most things, and I didn't want to completely shock her system, so I started small, with two drops, twice a day.

It's been eight days, and there's already a noticeable difference! The oil seems to tell her brain, "you're not in danger. Everything is okay. Take a nap." And when she's calmer, the whole pack is calmer. For Chesney, this is pretty miraculous.

We were out the other day, and normally, she'd be anxious. She saw a couple different dogs and heard them barking, and she let out just one bark. No panting, pacing, or going crazy. And in a new, unfamiliar spot with lots of smells of dogs, that was huge for her. I also took her home to see my parents recently, and she was much calmer with the CBD oil. She didn't even bark at the neighbors!

Before the CBD, I literally couldn't leave her alone because of her barking and anxiety. And now, I can calm her with the CBD before I leave! I've been going to Pilates for a couple of hours at a time. I have my life back. I'm not a slave to my dog anymore!

My only regret is not starting earlier. It makes a world of difference. The investment is totally worth it. We will never go without CBD again."

Chico, Mello, Moxie try CBD for Anxiety Relief

"I strongly believe in the power of CBD oil for people and pets. I have known about it for many years through watching documentaries about it and seeing it work wonders on people and pets. I have been an animal rescue volunteer for a long time, so I know firsthand just how miraculous it can be."

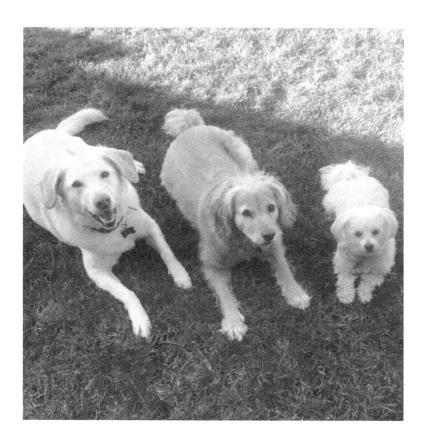

"As for my personal dogs, my 2-year-old Yorkie Poo Chico was already on CBD when I took him on as a foster in August of 2018. He was my first direct experience with using it on pets. He was dubbed "Little Cujo" by the rescue because he had severe anxiety about so many things.

Separation from me was the main one, but he was also territorial and possessive over me. If someone just stood next to me, he would go into attack mode. He also didn't like people touching him at all or getting too close.

So he came to me having just started CBD, and I continued it. I gave it to him every day. I started by giving the lowest recommended dose, but found I had to increase it quite a bit to get results. After about a month, there was a noticeable difference.

In fact, the other volunteers in the rescue were shocked at how far he had come. He could be touched, groomed, and picked up. I have now stopped giving it to him daily, and just save it for situations when he really needs it. It's definitely helped, although, I would like to see even more of an impact.

For example, he still growls at my larger male dog, Mello, for no reason. And if someone accidentally bumps him, it sends him into a frenzy. The oil I have been using is full spectrum hemp, but I'm going to try some with THC next to see if I can get different results. I want to be able to do things like take him to the vet without huge problems.

I give CBD to my other dogs, Mello and Moxie, as well. Mello is a seven-and-a-half-year-old yellow lab who I've had since puppyhood who is terrified of fireworks.

Before CBD, whenever there was fireworks, he wouldn't be able to settle down. He would pace, couldn't find a place that would make him feel secure, and he tried to calm himself by pressing his head against the wall, but nothing worked at all. "

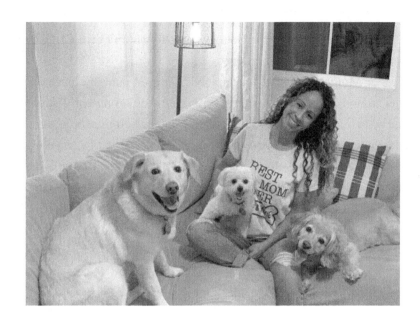

"Moxie is 6. She's a spaniel-retriever mix I've had since 1. She's back and forth. She's not as anxious as Chico or Mello, but she struggles with stranger anxiety. She settles better with CBD and warms up faster within one visit and doesn't bark like crazy like she used to.

And these aren't the only success stories I know. I spread the word about CBD to all my rescue people and everyone I know who has pets struggling. I gave some to friend who has a dog with cancer, and it improved his appetite.

The reason I bought some for myself years ago to begin with was because my rescue friend in the Bahamas had a dog who had seizures and had a miraculous recovery on CBD. His seizures virtually stopped. I know of volunteers who gave some to shelter dogs on 4th of July to help them cope. CBD is just powerful stuff. It's all-natural and just so, so helpful. "

Emily Brizon, Pet Nutritionist tries CBD for her 2 dog's anxiety and inflammation issues

"I have two Chows: Momo and Naga; to whom I give CBD, and they both do extremely well on it.

For Momo, we use it for anxiety. She used pant and pace when she was around a lot of new people or in a new environment. I started with one or two drops daily, about 10 to 15 minutes before people were due to come over or before we'd go to a new place that was going to be crowded, and the results were dramatic. Naga doesn't have issues with anxiety, but I still give him CBD as well for the overall health benefits.

I add it to both of their meals that I make at home to balance them out. It's got a lot of omega-3 and 6 fatty acids, which is excellent for them! When we were feeding them commercial food, a lot of oil built up on their coats, and they always needed baths. Now their skin and coats are healthy and soft and we take a lot longer between baths, thanks to the CBD.

As a pet nutritionist, I highly recommend CBD when I'm working with clients whose pets have the same coat issues. I like it better than fish oils because it's more sustainably harvested and you don't get the heavy metal contamination that you do with fish oil.

I especially like the CBD hemp oils because you get the full spectrum benefit. They often come in easy to ingest carrier oils such as coconut, avocado, or olive. Plus, a little goes a long way, which is nice. Using CBD hemp oil saves me money over the fish oil option, so it's been really great."

Danielle gives Charlie and Pablo CBD for Anxiety and Arthritis Pain.

"I've been a fan of CBD for years. I first learned about it through my local dispensary and was on board when it became available for pets about five years ago. I bought one of the very first Pet CBD Meds on the market for one of my senior dogs who has since passed Now I give it to both of my remaining seniors and sometimes my whole pack for various things. Anxiety? CBD. A little sore? CBD. Having trouble sleeping? CBD. Natural, safe and effective is my jam for my whole family.

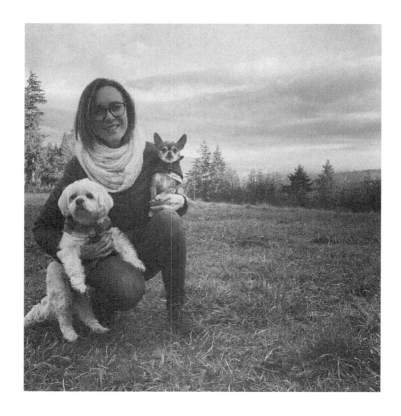

The dogs I mainly give it to now, Charlie--a Lhasa Apso--and Pablo--a Chihuahua--get it on a regular basis to treat their age-related conditions like anxiety and arthritis. I just mix it in with their dinner each night. "

"I also make my own dog treats and I like to put some oil in the treats (we give them away to our doggie friends, and they LOVE them, too)! Charlie and Pablo are also both on an assortment of medications as well as the CBD oil and get a healthy, vegan diet.

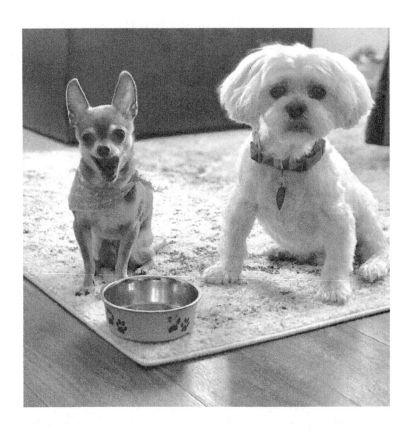

When I first started them on CBD regularly, I noticed differences gradually, but at two weeks, we were taking longer walks, running a little more, and sleeping a little better.

The CBD really helps them with anxiety and pain levels, so it allows me to keep their medication doses low. I would much rather give them natural CBD oil rather than higher doses of the heavy pharma meds they have to take already. In my experience, CBD has all the calming and healing effects that it advertises; I also take it myself! "

"I used to own a dog boarding facility and would advocate for CBD oil a lot to my clients; most everyone's experience was the same- those that thought the CBD wasn't helping didn't notice any negative side effects, and those who noticed it was helping didn't see any drawbacks.

It seemed to either work for them or it did nothing. In simple terms: it's totally harmless either way.

Charlie is particularly high maintenance...I can't leave him alone, I need to walk him in a stroller if we're going more than a couple blocks, and he is a 24/7 job...but I wouldn't change it for the world. I'll be right here carrying him up the stairs and walking him at 2am and giving him all the CBD treats and veggies he wants (he loves tomatoes the most)!

And Pablo is still kickin' for the most part...his knees are a little clicky now and then and he's got that grandpa cough, but he's still lead security for our pack and protecting all of us with all his five-pound might!

Me and my boys love being lazy together. We're old (ok, I'm 30-they're old) and we're tired and just happy being cozied up together with our cat. In the summer, we love beach days. Pablo stays guard by me while Charlie likes to lay at the water's edge and catch the waves that just touch the shore...he likes a cool belly.

We like to hang with our dog friends and go to grandma's and in the summer, we like to take long, slow walks and sniff everything. And naps. Naps are one of our favorite things, too. All of this is possible because CBD helps me manage their pain and health in a way that keeps them vibrant and loving life, even at their advanced ages.

I am an advocate for the cannabis industry and I think CBD is an important, integral, and wonderful part of this multi-dimensional plant. When it first came out, I was really excited to have my dogs try it. I've been happy with the results, and so have they!

If you're thinking about it for your pets, I encourage you to go for it! In my experience, they get all the benefits or nothing happens at all. There are no side effects or anything. There's nothing to lose and a ton to gain! If you're nervous about giving it to your pet, I'd just say...take it for yourself!"

Carson & Tanner's Anxiety vs CBD

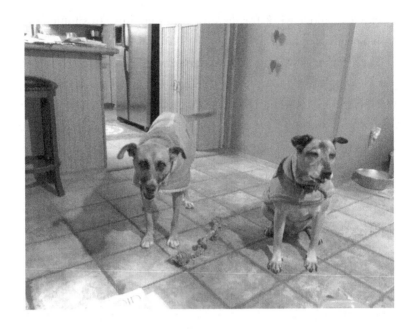

Tanner and Carson

"I have a 13-year-old rescue dog named Tanner who was severely abused. He came to me with many problems, and now 9 years later, Tanner is still full of anxiety and separation issues. He never liked to be away from me, and loud noises always distressed him. 2 years ago, though, it got a lot worse. On top of his regular separation anxiety, he started to get another type of anxiety associated with early dementia called "Sundowners Syndrome".

Starting around 10 pm, he would pace, bang into the walls and doors and scratch on them to get out, and pant intensely. This would go on until about 4 am, when he would finally drop from being exhausted. I took him to my vet, and she put him on meds, but they made his condition worse. I knew that he (and I) could not go through this much longer. I wasn't getting any sleep either because I was up trying to calm him down throughout the night.

I stumbled upon CBD online. I, myself, don't take meds because I am so sensitive to them, so I'm always looking for other solutions and often turn to the web to find alternative methods. It was during my online research for myself that I read up on doggie dementia.

I found a website put up by another woman who also had a dog that was dealing with anxiety, sundowners, and dementia, and she started to treat her dog with CBD oil with success. I started researching different companies and brands, and I finally ordered a bottle of CBD oil.

The first night I gave Tanner 18 drops on the tongue. He still had an episode, but it was not as bad. Every night I gave him some, and within days, I could see him being a little calmer and our nights were getting better.

When he started to get anxious from noises like thunder when it rained, I'd give him a few drops. I was also having a difficult time finding food he could and would eat. So I started to cook for him, and gradually added his dog food back in. The hemp helped his appetite and nausea as well. He was eating and keeping it down.

I notice that now, it's 2 years later, and I have reduced the amount he gets to maybe a few drops at night. Tanner has gotten so calm and relaxed since he's been on it, and it seems the hemp has built up in him, as he hardly needs it now. I noticed during the last thunderstorm, he didn't get excited and slept thru it.

It's just nice that I have a way to give Tanner a better quality of life, especially in his late years. He still loves being lazy at home and doesn't really like going places, but he still enjoys his daily car rides. My husband Nick and I load up both dogs every morning for a 15-mile drive that we all love."

I don't know what our outcome would of been if I hadn't have looked into hemp. Recently, I've started to give my other dog, Carson, a few drops two times a day for a muscle pull, and I can see the improvement. I have also recommended it to some of my friends and they, too, can't believe what a difference it has made".

Nala takes down Anxiety

"A little over a year ago, my 10-year-old Pomeranian-Poodle mix, Nala, started throwing up bile, had diarrhea, and was very lethargic. They diagnosed her with pancreatitis and started her on a short-term course of antibiotic and anti-inflammatory. She was also on a long-term course of probiotics and omega-3s. She did a little better on all of this, but not great.

She was still vomiting and very lethargic. Then she started having accidents in the house, so we had to confine her to the kitchen when we left for work, which she did not like at all. And then she stopped eating altogether. If dogs with pancreatitis don't eat on a regular basis, they throw up bile and the pancreas starts digesting itself. It's extremely important to make sure she eats, so we had to hand-feed her. My husband and I were taking turns doing it twice a day.

She also started obsessively licking. She was licking the air, licking her limbs. It caused her fur to mat and it also made her smell terrible. So we took her back to the vet and they said it was due to anxiety and recommended that she go on steroids, which I wouldn't do because she already wasn't feeling good, and steroids have a tremendous amount of side effects. So they put her on an allergy medication instead. It helped with the licking, but did not address any of the other problems.

Then one day, I was talking to my physical therapist about CBD. And all of a sudden, it dawned on me that maybe I should try it on Nala, so I researched pancreatitis in dogs and CBD oil. Unfortunately, there are no studies, but there are testimonials, so I read those. I also learned how to tell if CBD oil is good or not.

I saw Pets Strong CBD in a local pet boutique and looked up the details online. It met all the criteria: manufactured in the United States, organically farmed, and it had third-party lab results that you can actually view online. I bought it because--truthfully--my husband and I were at our wit's end, especially with all the hand-feeding. Once we gave it to her, I was expecting fast results, but she didn't make a very quick turnaround. Some people out there notice results in a day. Not us. It took a couple of weeks before we started to see huge improvement.

The biggest thing is her appetite improved. We no longer had to coax her to eat and hand-feed her! She was excited about meals again! And eventually, she stopped having accidents in the kitchen, so we gave her access once again to the whole house.

And she stopped licking, so then took her off her allergy medication too. So essentially, we've now taken her off everything. We went from spending about $150 per month on meds and vet visits to about $40 per month for the CBD. It's a huge relief. She's not so anxious, and she's active again! We call her "our little miracle." We can't believe it.

Other people have noticed, too. Our neighbors say she seems like a different dog. And I could only attribute it to the CBD oil that we've religiously given her twice a day for nine months. She will have a vomiting episode every once in a very great while, but that's it.

To other pet owners considering CBD, I suggest you start with a low dose and see what happens. You will most likely have to play around to find the right dose. Be patient. Don't expect that one dose is going to cure them. It's like any other kind of medication--you have to build it up in their body.

Until that happens, you're going to see improvement. But the process is certainly worth it, especially when your pet's quality of life is poor, and you just want to find a solution. I'm a pharmaceutical rep, so I have seen the investment in the process pay off time and again.

And I would say, once you start your pet on it, don't suddenly take them off their other meds; just gradually reduce the doses of whatever else they are on, and just see how they do until hopefully you can wean them off completely.

Finally, make sure you're getting a quality product. Obviously, we love Pets Strong. We've recommended it to other people. And if me telling my story helps one dog have an improved quality of life, I think that'd be fantastic, because it sure improved Nala's (and all of our) quality of life. I mean, I was so mad and upset with the whole situation at one point, I was ready to give her away because I just could not take it anymore. But now, she's just our lovable little puppy. If you are out there struggling too, there's no reason to be upset. Try CBD. Hopefully your life will improve as much as ours have!"

Rescue Black Lab Finds Peace from Anxiety

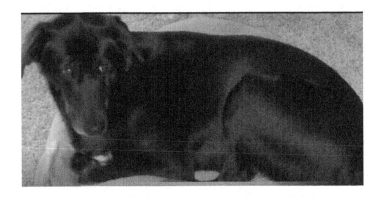

"We have a rescue dog. She is a black lab mix, 10 years old. She came to us with fear and anxiety; constantly pacing and would just hide in a corner and stay there and wouldn't come out, especially if men came over that she didn't know. New experiences for her, she would just close up and she would try to go hide somewhere under the bed or in a corner.

I learned about the CBD from my favorite dog trainer. She recommended giving it a try to see if it would help with her anxiety, and after about two weeks, I started noticing a difference.

We had somebody come over that she didn't know and she just went right up to him. She was not pacing around. Her tail was wagging. It was like she was excited to be part of the group, instead of going running off and hiding, which was a big breakthrough for her. CBD has really, really helped her come out of her shell. It's just been nice for her to be able to be a part of our family more, and it's just been a lot more fun to have her around."

Chapter Six
Arthritis in Pets and CBD Pet Parent Stories

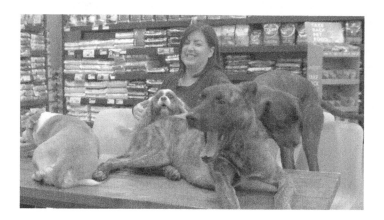

Gizmo tries CBD for hip discomfort

"We adopted Gizmo at age 10 from a local shelter. We don't really know his background, but based on exams and x-rays, the shelter determined that he had some arthritis, was kind of painful in the backend, and had potential neurological issues. Mostly, he just seemed really stiff and didn't want to move around a whole lot.

We first addressed his diet and hip pain, hoping that everything else would kind of fall into place. We looked for homeopathic solutions that would be easy for his older body to process. "

"We had had him about a month when we first discovered CBD oil. I didn't know much about it, but a friend of ours started using it for his dog. She is really anxious around new people, other dogs, and new spaces. They noticed a big difference, which was intriguing for us.

Plus, we heard that it was a nice multi-purpose holistic solution, as opposed to the prescription meds that can cause major issues with organs. Gizmo being a senior means it's kind of about quality of life over quantity, but we'd like to give him both. Why give him something that might be hard on his body if we don't have to?

We started with .5 mgs twice a day. Within the first week, his eyes seemed a little bit brighter. He seemed a little bit more tolerant of being more active throughout the day. But over the course of the past several months, he's become a lot more active. His appetite has become a lot more voracious.

Before, he would leave food and graze throughout the day. He was more of a free feeder, which didn't really work with our other two dogs. Now he actually joins the rest of the pack and eats twice a day--and eats his whole meal sometimes before the three-year-old dogs do! And he wants to play! He tries to play fetch. It's only about 3 feet, but he makes a good effort. He puts his best forward.

We give him one dose every day in his food, usually in the morning just so that he can get going. It's like his morning coffee, if you will. It gets him right for the day, and peps him up.

We experiment with it, so if we know that we're going to have a little bit more of an active day, we might give him a bigger dose. Or if we unintentionally had a really active day, we might give him an additional dose in the evening, so that he can at least feel a little better while he's recovering during his sleep.

Gizmo is a dog who a lot of people would have written off, thinking, "Oh, he has arthritis," and not believe he could have better or more. But with CBD, we were able to bring him back from the brink. Before, he would just sort of sit there and stare at us. He's been on CBD a little less than a year now, and it's been great. He definitely has become a lot more interested in affection and engagement--even demanding it sometimes! Plus, he's got a little sass back now, which is really nice to see"

Delilah, a 14 year old Pitbull tackles bad hips with CBD

"Our pittie Delilah is the oldest in our current pack. She's about 14 or so, and is the biggest, cuddliest dog baby you've ever met. She loves to hug and be with humans. She's our first pit bull, and she totally won us over (we had been small dog people before). She is just so sensitive and emotional, and it's really a shame pit bulls get such a bad rap.

Early on, our vets helped us determine that she was born with bad hips. Instead of a regular ball and socket with ligaments, Delilah's x-rays showed her sockets were nearly flat, and her bones were practically rubbing on each other. Her right side was worse than her left, so her orthopedic surgeon did a procedure on that one first, in 2016. Our plan was to go back and do the left side, too, but we never did."

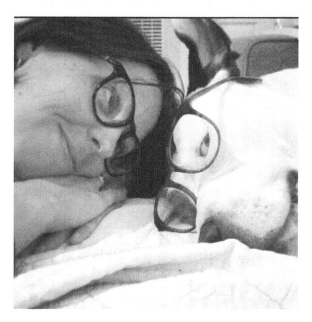

"She did great after the surgery--in fact, she came running out of the hospital! It was unlike anything I expected! We had to keep her quiet for 6 weeks post-op so she could recover properly, and it was a challenge. It still makes me laugh to remember how it didn't phase her at all.

So now it's 2019, and she's getting pretty old and stiff. The vets always told us to expect arthritis, even with the surgery. She started showing stiffness, refusing to go on walks, and having trouble getting up and down off the floor and up onto furniture about a year and a half ago.

We have been managing the pain with various pain meds and supplements off and on, but we haven't really found her magic combination yet. The other thing she's starting to show signs of is sundowners and early dementia, so now we have added CBD in to try to address both the arthritis and her mental and emotional distress.

We've known about CBD for several years. Being out in California, it's very common for people to use it on themselves and pets. We used it on another one of our dogs, Kali, last year during her final weeks to help ease her end of life transition, and it helped keep her calm.

We've been dosing Delilah with it for a few weeks now. It definitely has given her improved energy during the day. She is still stiff, but going on much longer walks (made it an hour the other night!), and is even playing again! And when we give it to her in the evening, it is helping to get her settled.

The only thing is, we haven't found her exact sweet spot with the ratio and dosage yet. Too little, and she's still agitated and painful. Too much, and she gets knocked out for like 15 hours. But we are on the road.

I think CBD is such a helpful tool, if you take it slow and understand it might take a little while to find the right product and dosage. I'm so glad it's becoming a more mainstream way to treat pets. I know we are looking at the last year or two of Delilah's life, which breaks my heart. But having CBD to help her is a huge relief to us all."

Fella and Aging Aches

My dog, Fella, is 12. I've had dogs my entire life, and he's by far the kindest, most gentle soul I've known. His heart is so pure. He and I have always had a special bond over running since he's a whippet. Now that he's a senior with arthritis and degenerative disc disease, our running days are over, but we still have fun together, and he's still loving life. That wasn't always the case, though.

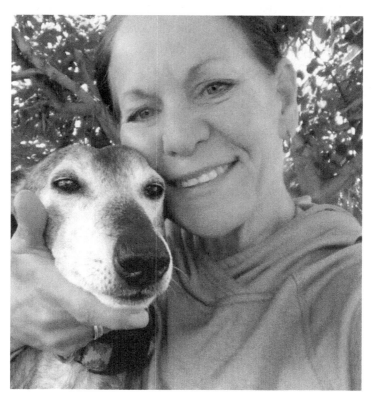

5 years ago, I gave him a dose of Trifexis for flea and tick control. Immediately afterwards, he had a seizure and fell. Ever since that, his body and mind haven't been the same. The seizure caused a lot of damage. He was stiff and scared and even stopped walking for awhile. Once he healed from initial fall, he could walk again, but about a year

later, he began having intense pain. He started crying when he moved and in the middle of the night from pain. I took him to the vet for a full assessment. The x-rays showed degenerative disc disease.

They put him on Gabapentin and Carprofen. I added in some supplemental chondroitin and glucosamine. I also took him for hydrotherapy, cold laser treatments, and massage. The hydrotherapists were the ones who suggested CBD for him. At that time, it was hard to find, and my choices were limited.

The original capsules and cookies didn't do much. But about two years ago, my friend became a distributor of a very high quality oil, which I tried, and it made a huge difference.

Within a few days, it seemed to calm the inflammation. And he was able to go on longer walks. After his seizure, he had also become very jumpy and skittish, and Rescue Remedy just wouldn't help. The CBD, however, calmed his stress as well.

For about the past year now, he's been virtually pain and symptom-free. He doesn't take anything now; only if he's having flare up. He's so much more active and has a zest for life again. It's really remarkable. I mean, there was a point where his pain was so unmanageable,

I was considering putting him down because his quality of life was so bad. Now, he's like a whole different dog. He's balanced and moves well. Knowing he is virtually pain-free now is a major relief and joy to me. To have this extra time with my kind-hearted sage is a gift. And it's not just extra time; it's extra GOOD time.

Charley and Arthritis Pain

Charley is our nine-and-a-half-year-old Collie mix and loves hiking! Our lives pretty much revolve around being outside and trekking our favorite nearby trails. But about six months ago, I took Charley into the vet because she had become stiff and was limping after our walks. She also started crying out in pain when I'd get up from her bed. This was no good for a dog who loves to be active. I set out to figure out what was going on and how I could help Charley.

46

The vet diagnosed Charley as having arthritis in her left hip and recommended Meloxicam for the pain. Before I started actually treating Charley with it, I spoke to a few people who had their dogs on the same medication.

Ultimately, I decided that I didn't like how hard that drug was on their organs and I also didn't like the list of potential side effects. It just seemed like a last line of defense; not something to use coming through the starting gate. I wanted to find an alternative that wouldn't put Charley at so much risk for organ failure and other problems.

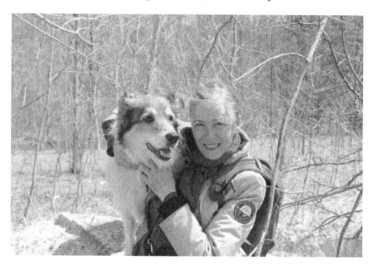

I was already well aware of CBD before Charley's diagnosis because a friend of mine makes CBD oil for humans and pets, and had been treating a dog in my building for debilitating seizures. I knew she'd been seizure-free for 6 months, so I approached him to ask about treating Charley's arthritis. He worked with me to start her on the correct dose, and nearly immediately Charley went from being a limping old lady to chasing squirrels in the ravine again. Today, Charley is doing wonderfully. She and I are back to our old hiking ways, enjoying all the outdoors has to offer!

Tashi and Arthritis Discomfort

When I was diagnosed with breast cancer in 2013, I started researching alternative treatments and supplements, and came across information about CBD. It helped me in my recovery, plus I also discovered it wasn't just helpful for people, but that it could work on pets too.

That came in handy when my dog Tashi started freaking out over fireworks that same year. The CBD worked like a charm on her to calm her down. She went from complete shakes and clinging, panting, not eating, and terror to taking herself into the bathroom, jumping in the tub, and nesting in there. She had never done that before. She tends to fall asleep eventually. That's her favorite safe spot now. She also still eats and take treats during fireworks, which is huge.

But then she started getting older, and with her age came back and joint problems. She's about 11 or 12, and about 3 years ago, she was diagnosed with arthritis and lumbar inflammation. I was away when Tashi had her first major episode. She got really bad diarrhea and couldn't control her bowels. X-rays showed that her lumbar region was inflamed and pressing on the nerve/muscle that controlled her bowels, so we had to get solutions fast. She was diagnosed with arthritis on the spot. It showed up in her hips too. That was May 2016.

The vet prescribed Rimadyl, and it did help; however, I didn't feel that this was a long-term option for pain and inflammation management. There are just far too many side effects and vet visits involved, so I immediately looked to CBD for long-term treatment.

It took a few tries to find the exact product that worked for Tashi. I had a lot of confusion about the THC-based carrier and full-spectrum hemp and isolate. Cost has also been an issue for me in the past; however, I found a company that offers a deep discount to veterans, disabled, and low-income people. They also have great pet products, so that was very helpful in making CBD more affordable to Tashi and me. Full-spectrum hemp CBD has worked best for me personally, and I don't worry about THC overdosing, and that's what has worked for Tashi too.

If she had something more serious, I would look into a THC option, though.

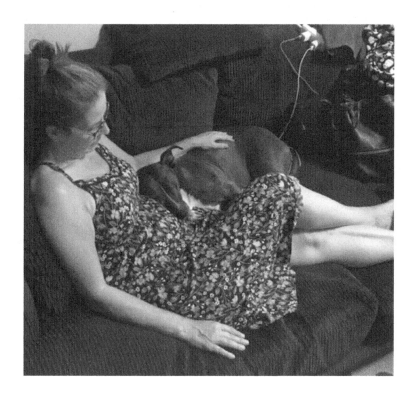

I put it on her food morning and night, and she likes it. Occasionally, I buy her CBD treats, too--when I find them on sale--and she loves those! Once I found what she liked dialed in the right dosage, I was able to see results within a few days! She was instantly more relaxed and pain-free. Today, she's doing so well. You wouldn't even know she had issues-- she's playful and active, and romps around!

I mean, this dog is just so resilient. She lost an eye to cancer in 2019 and continues to be the same food motivated, tummy rub-loving, skateboard-hating dog she's always been. She still loves life as much as ever. My favorite thing to do with her is to take her on car rides and watch the sheer joy she has when she realizes we are gong in the car.

Seeing CBD work so well for her over the years--especially on her back--makes me feel good about treating her with natural products, and I know that long-term, she will have better health and quality of life.

Chapter Seven

Skin & Coat Inflammation & Severe Itching in Pets Pet Parent CBD Stories

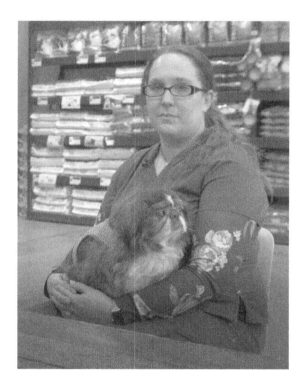

Torque Tries CBD for Skin Inflammation

"I rescued Torque when he was nine months old. At that point, he had been locked in a basement for about five months. He was covered in his own filth, and I don't know what kind of nutrition he was getting.

A lot of these dog health issues start in puppyhood and stem from poor nutrition. So when I got him, I put him on a good food and so on, but he still struggled with chronic ear infections, skin infections, and skin mites. I noticed that every issue [he] was having was somewhere related to an inflammation of the skin or in his intestines. The vet prescribed antibiotics and steroids, which would help for a little bit, but it would start up again and become a cycle. Eventually, he started forming scar tissue in his ear canals because of the chronic infections.

He is also a competitive dock diver, so in addition to the pain, I couldn't have a dog with sores competing in water, so it was quite challenging. It was a constant struggle. I also discovered that any time he had any kind of a high-stress situation happen, these skin infections would just explode, almost like an auto-immune response.

It eventually got to the point where all four paws were infected, and it was both fungal and bacterial, in different combinations on all four paws. So the vet was putting him on heavy doses of antibiotics and anti-fungals, 30 days at a time, several times per year. That's a lot of times to wipe his gut bacteria.

So then, a turning point happened recently where Torque ate something he shouldn't have and had to go to the ER. His stomach was pumped, he received activated charcoal treatments, injections, medications...all this stuff. Right after that, His paws just exploded. They were literally oozing, they were so bad.

And then a friend recommended CBD, but I was like, "well, he doesn't have anxiety." But she told me that it works throughout the body--there are so many receptors for CBD, and the skin and immune system is part of it.

So I tried it. I stopped shampooing and spraying his paws with the medications and applying salves, which he would scream and fight me on the whole time, anyway, and just made his stress worse.

What was really shocking to me was that within days, I could notice a significant decrease [of the irritation and infection on his paws]. And within a week, there were only small spots of red here and there. And now--they look amazing! His front right paw looks better than it ever has--there's literally no red! I can't get over that. A few drops nightly is all it takes. No more pills or creams or sprays. It's been an absolutely incredible experience!

I will say, the only thing that scares me is he knows it comes in a glass bottle with a dropper, and he goes crazy for it, so I have to keep it up. He grabbed another bottle thinking it was the CBD and crushed it! Luckily, it wasn't anything poisonous. But he loves it, which I know is not always the case, but it makes it a lot easier for us. It also makes it easier financially to have just one substance, instead of the seven or eight different things to treat him. CBD has really been a life-changer for him and me!"

Delvina Finds Relief From Severe Itching

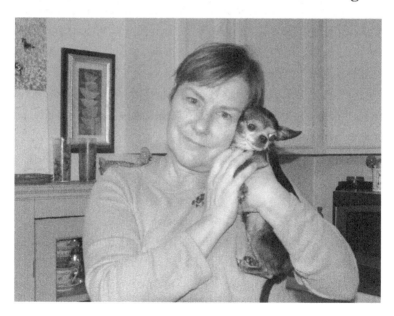

"Delvina is an eight-year-old Teacup Chihuahua. And about two years ago, she developed a problem with itching and she would scratch herself so badly that she had scabs and scratches all over her neck and she was starting to lose hair on her hunches and her lower back because she was biting at herself.

We took her to the vet thinking she have a bad case of mites or fleas. But nothing like that showed and vet diagnosed her with an allergic reaction. So we went through the whole protocol for allergy problems and tried different proteins. No matter what we did, she still constantly itched.

So after the vet wasn't able to help us, we tried some natural things. A friend of mine told me about CBD and I have bought and tried a CBD oil and it did not helped Delvina at all. Little did I knew at that time that not all CBD products were created equal and there are unfortunately lot of bad companies out there just selling hemp oil as CBD.

But I had the bottle already bought so I tried increasing the dose. That did not work at all either. And so we tried some other natural remedies but nothing was having an impact to help Delvina.

And so a couple of months ago, we were discussing actually putting her to sleep, because we felt she was suffering so much, and a friend of mine brought up CBD again, and I told her I didn't even want to try it, because it didn't work before and she said, "Well, this is a different company, it's called Pets Strong, and I really believe in these people that they're doing something really good and they have a really amazing product. I've actually seen it work on my dog."

And so I tried it. The very first day we started giving it to her she itched less. The second day we gave it to her I don't think she itched at all. And I found that with the dog that size that they need to have a dose more frequently than larger dogs, because of their metabolism. So she gets a dose four times a day of just a few drops of the Pets Strong CBD oil and she has no problems anymore with itching.

I will add however when I have noticed that the people that don't notice a huge significant change in their dog after tying CBD, may be it is because their dog is not on a healthy diet or they're not really being consistent with giving them the drops. Like any wellness routine, you cant try CBD once in a while.

But I think it's good for all dogs. I think it would benefit any animal, whether it's a dog or a human being or a cat to take this oil. It's very high in omega-3, and it's got the cannabinoids, like our systems have and it resonates with us and it's very good for us and so it's good for any pet, even if they don't have a problem, it would be healthy for them."

Junior Finds His Love of Kids Again

"I have a Jack Russel. His name is Junior. He's 11 years old. He started having health problems about two years ago. He had growths on his back. He was having problems with his hips. He was losing his hair. We tried different treatments. We tried changing his food. Nothing we did worked.

We started the CBD oil and within a week we noticed a huge difference. His hair wasn't growing back yet. It took about probably two weeks before that started growing back, but he stopped itching and scratching and he was in a, definitely, in a better mood.

He's a very lovey dog, generally, but you couldn't get near him. He would bare his teeth because he was in pain. He was hurt and he was itchy. He just did not want to be bothered.

Even with my kids, he would go lay with my kids and they would just move his feet around and he would growl and bare his teeth. After CBD, he is no longer doing them. I heard about CBD being used for humans. I never really thought about it using it for a dog and it's just, it's been a godsend. He's is acting like he is five years younger."

Chapter Eight

Leuk's Landing: Helping Cats with Feline Leukemia

By Leona Foster, Founder

I run Leuk's Landing, which is a sanctuary for cats that have feline leukemia, and we have been using CBD for our cats with great success. Feline leukemia is a disease that's always fatal. Cats infected with it don't live beyond maybe 6 years--as opposed to a cat without it that would live to be 20. The only thing you can really do for a cat who has it is provide what the vets call "supportive care"--that is, boosting their immune systems since theirs is compromised.

About four years ago, I read that CBD has the power to do just that. Plus, it can help with some of the other issues our cats face--like anxiety and pain--so I started working with a CBD company that provides me with capsules that we have used off and on in a variety of situations. It's turned out to be particularly helpful with pain management. The human crisis with opioids has now invaded the veterinary world, and it's extremely difficult to get any amount of pain medicine for cats. So we use CBD instead.

One very memorable instance was about three years ago with one of our cats named Leo. A tumor started growing in one of his eyes. We had him on the normal course of steroids, which is used often for inflammation, but it didn't seem to be working, so I tried CBD. And we noticed very quickly that the tumor started shrinking until it was gone. In the end, the tumor did come back, but the CBD gave him probably another six good months of life that he wouldn't have had.

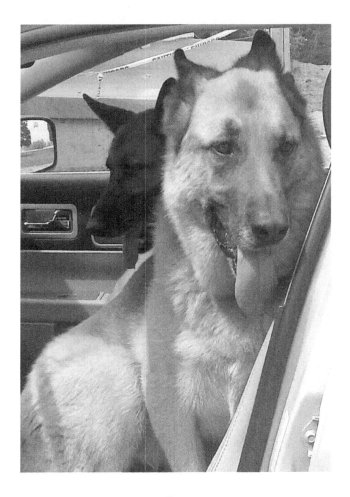

Rex

Currently, I'm using CBD on two cats. One of them--Sky--has some type of irritable intestinal issue. We've had her on steroids, and she has been doing okay, but I decided maybe we should give CBD a try. It's been three weeks now, and she seems much perkier, she's gaining some weight back, and overall her fur quality, her appetite...everything seems much improved.

Then there's Bran. He's about nine months old. Around the same time about I started with Sky, I decided, "what the heck, let's give him some of the CBD too" because he was very skinny. One of the things with this leukemia is that their muscle tone atrophies and their appetite wanes quite a bit. But he's been doing extremely well on the CBD. He looks good, and his high fever has been down. He's eating extremely well, and his eyes just look much improved; you can see that he feels better. So right now he is maintaining. This is the first time I've gone down this path, but so far, I can say historically, he should not still be with us based on where he was. I don't know what more time he'll have, but at the moment he's doing quite well.

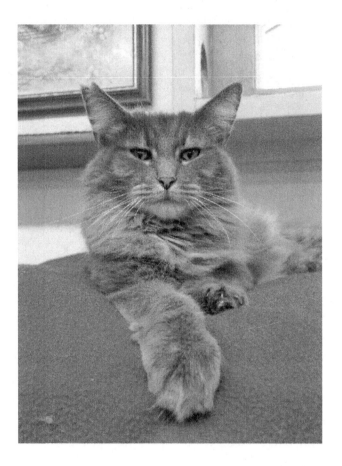

Sky

In addition to it working with my cats, I bought CBD for my mother's German Shepherd that had the classic German Shepherd hip dysplasia and severe arthritis. It was amazing to see him going from having a very difficult time walking to doing much, much better within about two weeks.

It seems like traditional western medicine has side effects, like causing diarrhea or other things. Once nice thing about CBD, it seems to not have any side effects--at least in these instances that I've run into.

Overall, I think CBD is fairly reasonably priced, and it's worth trying, particularly when you do your homework and you see the things that it's known to work with the most, like pain, arthritis, digestion, and anxiety. I don't think there's a lot to risk. And then you just have to be a bit patient waiting for it to kick in, just like anything else.

For more information and to donate please visit https://www.leukslanding.org.

Chapter Nine

Joint and Disc Pains in Pets
Pet Parent CBD Stories

Finding Franklin Happiness Again

"I adopted Franklin from my local shelter 10 years ago, when he was just a few months old. I met him when I was volunteering, and it was love at first sight. He was adorable and all scruffy. They said he was some sort of Dandie Dinmont mix. I didn't even know what kind of dog that was at the time. All I knew is that he was a baby, he was sick, and he was mine.

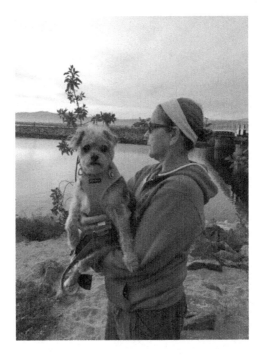

"He came home with some kennel cough, but we got that cleared up right away. He also came home with a much bigger health issue that we didn't fully understand until years later. They said he had come from a hoarding situation, and had a broken tail. They weren't sure how he had gotten it, but it didn't seem to bother him. You could tell by looking at it something was wrong--it just sort of hung limply without any control or movement--but other than that, it didn't seem to be an issue...until about four years ago.

That was when his personality changed. He went from being very social to being withdrawn. He started walking strangely--as though his rear end hurt. He was crying and whimpering, and was lethargic. We took him to the vet, and they suspected he had major inflammation and degeneration in his spine, possibly caused by his broken tail that went untreated for so long--but only because we didn't know it actually bothered him. The vet suggested we see a veterinary chiropractor, so we did, and he got acupuncture. We also took him to hydrotherapy. This all worked well for about two years, and that's when I heard about CBD.

I learned about it and started it for myself, actually, to treat joint pain, anxiety, and insomnia. I already knew about the benefits about smoking pot because my loved ones have treated themselves with it for Parkinson's. I also lived through the AIDS epidemic in the 80s, and lost a lot of friends to the disease. They often smoked it to ease their pain and sickness. But I'm not a smoker, so when CBD became an option, I was very interested and tried it. And it worked extremely well. I had been in and out of all sorts of treatments and had been taking drugs and supplements, but nothing worked like CBD. I was able to go from seeing my chiropractor once a week to once every couple of months! So I asked a holistic vet friend of mine what he thought about giving it to Franklin, and he said it was just starting to be used on pets with success, and I should try it for him. Sure enough--just as it did with me, it has kept him away from therapy. I give it to him orally and topically."

"He has been on pain meds in the past, but I just never really liked the side effects. He always seemed so out of it. His eyes were always glassy, he was lethargic, and just lost his zest for life. With CBD, we can keep his pain at bay without those side effects, and without constantly going to hydrotherapy. Actually, it's been two years since he's needed to be in the pool! And I have to admit, we've been out of CBD for a few weeks and I haven't had a chance with the busy holiday season to get more...and I can tell. His movement is bad again, and he's been whimpering. I need to get out there and get more, like, now!"

Fen & Degenerative Spine Disease Pains

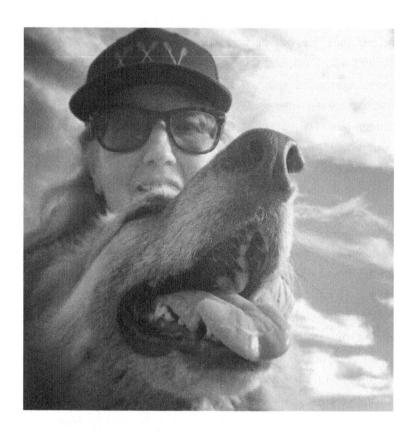

"Fen, my eleven-and-a-half-year-old Longhaired German Shepherd, has been on CBD for his arthritis and degenerative spine issues for about a month now. I adopted Fen when he was just a 14 week-old-puppy from a local shelter. He was very sick with mange and scabies, but I loved him immediately, and got him back to full health in no time.

Fast forward to 2017. That's when Fen began showing signs of arthritis and degenerative spine issues. He was having trouble with the stairs and walking any distance. He also started having trouble being able to control his bowels.

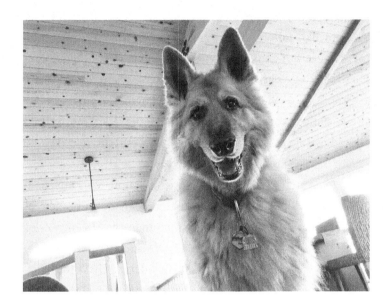

Fen's vet prescribed daily Gabapentin, which he still takes. Fen also started getting Adequan injections every 3 weeks about a year ago. He also had a prescription for Rimadyl, but I had been holding that in reserve for when he would eventually worsen and need something more down the road. I did the same with CBD. I knew all about it already because a lot of my friends had been using it successfully on their pets, and I wanted to use it as my final ace in the hole.

When I started CBD (and the Rimadyl) a month ago, the difference was nearly immediate. I saw results within about a week of starting, and he's still showing great improvement. There are no issues with the stairs, he's walking about a mile each morning and afternoon, having no accidents, and is chatty as ever! But just to make sure he's doing well and the meds aren't causing any other problems, I take him in for a senior blood panel every six months.

I give Fen .25ml of his tincture each morning with his food, which is the recommended dose according to his weight, with the ability to do it twice a day should I need to later on. Fen loves eating in general, so it's not been a problem to get him to take it.

I haven't noticed any negative side effects, but I love how much more engaged he seems! He's more chatty in the morning! Not so much barking; more like talking as we get ready for our morning walk, like "let's go!" He has full conversations trying to get me out the door!

Fen and his two-year-old Catahoula sister Bel are family members to me. Being able to see Fen doing so well, having so much energy, and enjoying his senior years means the world to me. We live in the country and walking together as a family is a huge part of our day that Fen doesn't have to miss now.

I know most pet owners fear adverse reaction with any pain relief product. When selecting a CBD product, I made sure she chose a reputable high-quality organic brand since there has been no definitive veterinary/scientific study done on how CBD affects pets.

My best advice to other pet owners considering CBD for their pets is to do the research and establish a direct contact with the company that makes the CBD. Look for a place that provides wonderful customer service and gives great advice on starting dosage and how you can increase it if you need to. The CBD company I work with even sent me an article about new research that made sense to them, and we adjusted Fen's dose accordingly. Love that!"

Charlie is Fetching Again

"My Corgi, Charlie, LOVES to play fetch. Frisbees are his favorite, but he'll chase anything. I've had him since he was just a puppy, and he's 13 now, and it's still the thing he lives for. 3 years ago, he blew out a knee chasing a tennis ball. He went for the ball, and then just stopped." "He wouldn't put weight on his leg at all. I knew something was seriously wrong. The vet said it was a clearly a tear that would need TPLO surgery. We had it done, and he did great and recovered fine. But a year later, he did it to his other knee, so he had to have another TPLO surgery on that one!

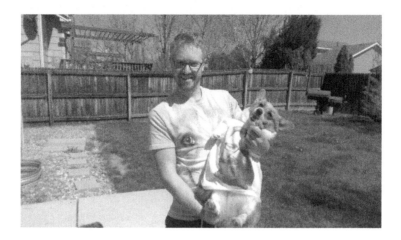

The surgeries were both successful and took away the pain he was experiencing, but after he fully recovered, when we would play fetch for long periods of time, his back legs would shake and he'd be more sensitive to walking on them. It just seemed like his joint pain was still flaring up after a lot of use. He loves playing so much that I hate taking fetch away from him because of his pain. But since I've never liked or used pharmaceutical pain meds for him, I haven't known what to do. I have tried to keep our fetch games short and limited, but he always wants more. So that's where CBD has come in.

The vet who diagnosed and treated Charlie the second time told me about it, but I didn't really consider it until I was in a place that sold CBD products a few weeks ago, and they had dog treats, so I figured I'd give it a try. It seemed to work after the first day I gave him a treat! He seemed a lot more comfortable after our fetch session! He didn't seem to be in the pain he usually is, and he was also a bit more relaxed overall, so that was a bonus.

It's been such a relief to see the impact it's having on his pain. I am more willing to play fetch with and for him longer since his knees don't seem to hurt him as much after. We are both much happier now that we have CBD in the mix and can play as much as he wants!"

Chapter Ten
Regaining Lost Appetite
Pet Parent CBD Stories

Lola Finds Her Appetite Again (and less anxiety)

"I have been giving CBD to my rescue cats, Lola (15 and a half years old) and Ollie (8 years old), since March 2018, and have seen great results. It started it originally because I wanted to treat Ollie for his behavior issues.

He used to compulsively lick himself and objects. It was so bad, he wore holes in rugs, couches, and even his own fur. He also was aloof and aggressive. I even had to separate him from Lola a lot because he attacked her. Everyone was stressed out. It felt ridiculous to have two small cats in a house with a baby gate. I also worried he would bite guests. He never wanted affection and rarely purred.

I visited the vet and they put him on Prozac originally, for about a year. It worked, but I hated giving it to him, hated going to the vet all the time for it, and I worried about the long-term effects. Also, he was loopy and zombie-like and eventually stopped eating the food I was hiding it in. I started researching alternatives online, and that's when I learned about CBD. I decided to ditch the Prozac completely and replace it with CBD oil capsules, which totally changed their lives.

Now Ollie is an affectionate, (still neurotic), funny, and sometimes really sweet cat. He sits on my lap! He loves being pet, which he never allowed before. I almost never have to separate him and Lola, which is so much easier. I am not sure CBD is the entire reason for this, but I do think his anxiety and fear has decreased a ton."

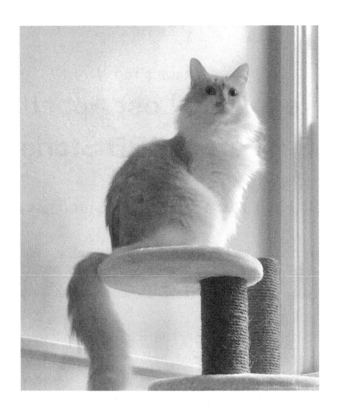

Ollie

"Around the same time of me giving it to Ollie for the first time, Lola was diagnosed with small mast cell cancer in her intestines and a cancer-like mass on her lung. When I got the diagnosis, I knew I would never treat it medically because

Lola is so traumatized by going to the vet. It just wasn't worth it to put her through it, especially at her older age. Instead, I put her on CBD too, not really knowing if it would do anything, but hoping to calm her a little bit through her final days and let nature take its course. But Lola and CBD had other plans.

After about a month, there was a big turnaround. At the time she was diagnosed, Lola was lethargic and looked terrible. I hoped the CBD would just ease any anxiety and possibly encourage her to eat…that was 18 months ago, and Lola's now back to eating, playing, and is stable!

Lola is my heart. She and I have been together for 15.5 years. So her being sick is like a gut punch. Today, she is running around yelling at me playing with toys...I spend every second I can with her, giving her my love and attention. I feel like CBD has given me these 18 additional months with her--and that's invaluable."

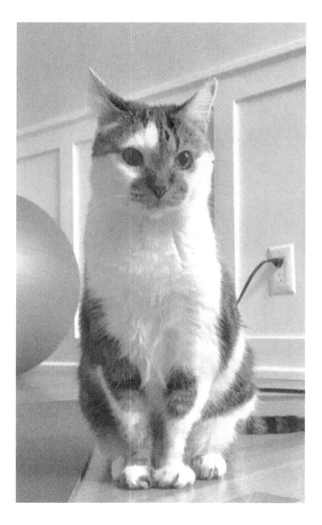

Lola

Trying CBD After Cancer Diagnosis

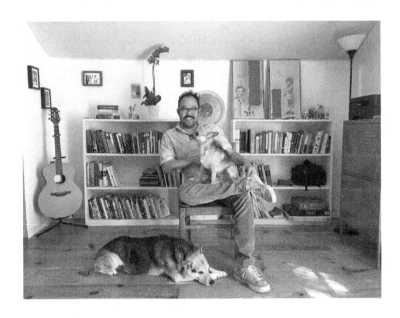

"I have two dogs, Tiki and Memo. In December of 2017, I got the most devastating news: my beloved 11-year-old German Shepherd/Huskie mix, Memo, had cancer.

I opted not to pursue chemo or radiation, but the vet did prescribe medications to manage the pain. They seemed to help a little, but not as much as I had hoped they would, so I turned to my big network of friends and contacts to see if they had any other ideas.

That's when I heard about CBD. At first, I was hesitant to try it. I equated it more with people smoking marijuana. I didn't understand the difference between CBD and THC. But over and over again, my friends encouraged me to try it for Memo, and since I wasn't totally impressed with what the pain medication was doing anyway, I gave it a shot.

I tried giving Memo CBD oil on a treat, which worked like a charm, and I think it only took about a day and a half before I saw it kick in. He was clearly not as painful. On the flip side, he was also sleepy and a little more lethargic than usual, but it was a small price to pay for the results.

Memo is still hanging in there! In fact, his pain is under enough control that I was able to stop giving him CBD, but I knows if he needs it again, CBD will always be an option. It gives me peace of mind knowing that I have a way to successfully manage his quality of life. I've been happy with what CBD has been able to do, and couldn't wish for more…except maybe if it kept Memo around forever? That'd be about it."

Alby Finding Balance with CBD

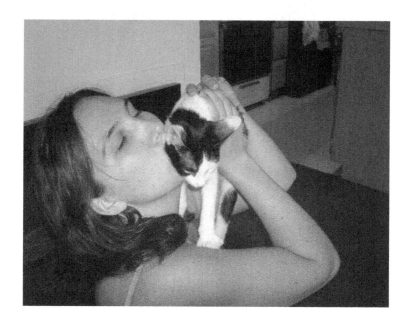

"My 12-year-old Tuxedo cat, Alby, has several health issues, including IBS, lymphoma, and leukemia, and we are currently integrating CBD with his traditional veterinary medicine.

He is on tons of medication, including pill chemotherapy that he gets once a month and we take him in for blood tests weekly. His first blood tests post-chemo showed that he is slightly anemic. The trouble is, they don't know if the anemia is from the chemo, or acid reflux from being on so many meds. He has a lot of trouble being interested in food…and even when he does try to eat, he has a hard time keeping it down. His stomach is really messed up from the cancer, plus all the medication.

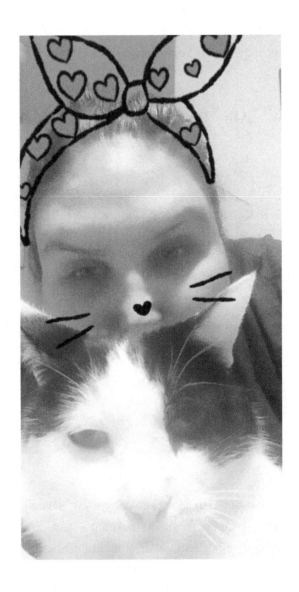

We've known about CBD for awhile--well before Alby's diagnosis--because both my husband and I have smoked marijuana for years; we both have medical cards in Illinois. Recently, we had been hearing more and more about CBD for dogs and cats. In fact, I foster for a rescue group here in Illinois, and they use CBD regularly to treat their rescue pets who have seizures, asthma, and other conditions. So we decided to try it for Alby.

We kept his vets informed and let them know we were going to add it into his regimen. They haven't really taken a position one way or another because they say there hasn't been enough research on it, but they certainly haven't discouraged us from giving it to him.

As soon as we started the CBD, Alby's nausea seemed to almost completely go away! He does get very sedated, though, which is fine with us because we know he isn't feeling well most of the time.

But the good thing is, lately, he does seem to have a little bit of energy returning and his lymph nodes have gone down. Also, the CBD has given him more of an appetite and he's eating like crazy (even though he hasn't gained any weight back yet)! This is a super hopeful sign, and something his other meds (even the anti-nausea ones) couldn't do.

He's also started laying with my husband and me and his brother again. He used to do it a lot before he got sick, but then stopped and wanted to be left alone. It's so nice to have him with us as a family!

He's also getting in boxes again, and cleaning himself again, which had stopped for awhile, even though he used to be obsessive about it. It's just basically like CBD is helping him get back to himself in a way the meds alone haven't been able to.

My heart bursts to see him returning to more of his normal behaviors, even though we know there's still a ways to go. Given how far he's come with the CBD in such a short amount of time, I'm very hopeful that Alby will be able to turn a few corners and keep his symptoms at bay for the long-term."

Luna Finds Her Appetite

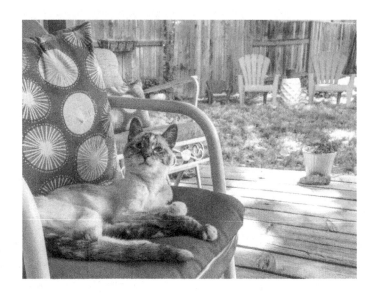

"I had my cat Luna for about 4 years. I rescued her from a little cat rescue in LA, and she's the cutest little Tortie-Siamese mix. About 6-8 months ago, she started vomiting, stopped eating, and began losing weight, and we don't know why.

She's now down to only 5 pounds, and we still don't really know what's wrong her. We've taken her to the vet, but because she's so small and too weak for true treatment, we aren't putting her through a big battery of tests. She's 12, so she's on the older side, too. We are guessing it's cancer, but don't know for sure. She's also on thyroid medication on top of this.

They've given her anti-nausea meds to try to stop her from vomiting, but they haven't worked at all, so about a week ago, I started giving her CBD. I've known about CBD for a long time in the human world, but I only recently learned that you can also give it to pets. At first, I was worried it might negatively impact her somehow, but I reasoned that she was already doing poorly, and we had possibly more to gain than lose at this point. This was kind of a last-ditch effort.

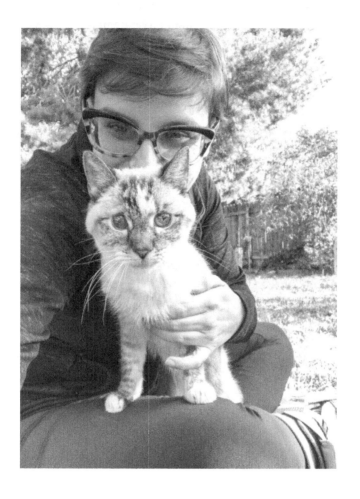

As soon as I started giving her the CBD, she stopped vomiting. It was actually pretty incredible to see how fast it worked! She seems a lot more comfortable and her stomach seems like it is settling. The only problem is, she's still not eating much. She is eating a little fresh salmon each day and I am syringe-feeding her some high-protein "recovery" food. Oh - and she eats organic whipped cream! But very little of each. Surprisingly, her energy is decent, though, for how little she eats. She's just skin and bones. Poor girl.

I don't know if we can beat this or get her to the point where she's actually increasing calorie-consumption and gaining weight, but we sure are trying. She is the best little cuddler, and I'm not ready to say goodbye quite yet. She's not puking anymore, so that's a huge step in the right direction, at least!"

Jupiter and Appetite Issues due to Cancer

"In September of 2019, my 14-year-old cat Jupiter stopped eating properly and started hiding from me. I have had him since he was 8 weeks old, and he had never done this, so I knew something was wrong.

When I took him to see the vet, they found a mass on his inner cheek and thought it was an ulcer from a rodent bite or something. They put him on antibiotics and prednisone, and he responded well at first, but we decided to test it just to be safe. It came back as squamous cell carcinoma (SCC), which he had before in his ear. He went in for removal three days later.

To help him with getting his appetite back and deal with the pain, I wanted to try CBD. Since CBD was legal here in Canada, I already knew what it did for humans, so I knew it had to do something for pets.

I had to wait a few days post-op because he didn't react well to the drugs they gave him in the hospital and he got so constipated. Once he pooped and no drugs were in his system, I gave him his first dose--this was about one or two weeks after his surgery.

I gave him human CBD hemp oil to start. I microdosed him and didn't notice anything, so then my friends suggested an oil with THC in it. I feared THC would hurt him. I cried so hard before giving him his first dose. I had friends talking to me and telling me I was doing the right thing. "

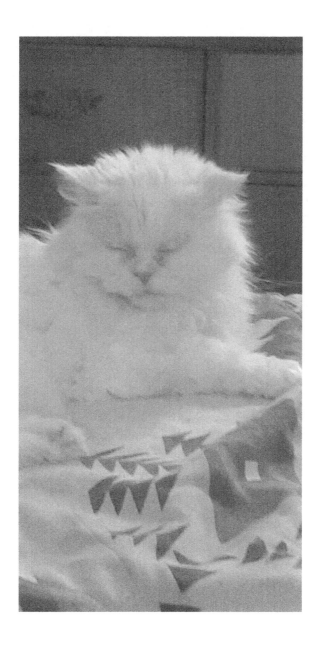

"We had all researched it, and new it would be okay, but I was still so nervous, I was shaking as I gave it to him. In a few days, he was more himself. His appetite came back with a vengance, he was more bouncy, and he was washing himself more. "

During his surgery, they got clean margins, but I can tell his mass is coming back because his gland is swollen. The good news is, that it's minor, and he doesn't know. SCC is so aggressive that it should have come back much sooner--like within weeks.

I had another kitty who had it in her gums. We removed it, and it came back three weeks later--and it was much worse. With Jupiter, I can tell it's there, but it's slow-growing. When I give him the CBD oil via syringe, I aim the oil at it, so he essentially gets it topically as well as orally.

He still has tons of energy, an amazing appetite and zero pain. He's doing so well and he's very healthy and happy. If it does grow back, I will have it removed again after Christmas because he's overall in great shape, and the mass is on his inner lip, so it's easy to remove.

I still worry about losing Jupiter too soon. I got him right after my first husband passed away. I named him after the song "Hey Jupiter" by Tori Amos, which was the last song my husband and I slow danced to. He always wanted a white cat, so I got Jup to honor him. Jupiter is my original grumpy cat.

He was born grumpy--he hates humans (except for me), but loves cats. He loves to put his face deep in the fur of other cats and snuggle. He is also a very spiritual cat. My current husband is Native, and Jupiter has appeared to him during the Sundance and sweat lodge. He has also visited my best friend during her meditation.

He's an amazing creature. He even had ear cancer and survived. I will do anything to save him, but now he is doing so amazingly well now on the CBD, so who knows how much more I will actually need to do. The CBD works better than any other meds out there we have tried.

Chapter Eleven
Candice Whitson
At Whits End Dog Training

"CBD has been a part of my personal and professional life for a while now. My husband, Matt, and I had looked into it a little bit for our son who has autism, but didn't do serious research until a rep from Pets Strong contacted our business about offering it, and we fell in love with the company. We're really proud to be able to offer something that is not only local, but all natural and done right.

Matt and I run At Whit's End Dog Training, based in Center Line, Michigan. We have been in business for a little over a year now. Matt had been training dogs for other people for about 11 years and decided that he wanted to do his thing.

Working for other companies ties your hands a little bit as to who you can help and how you can help, and he wanted freedom to do the right thing. Sometimes you have senior citizens or others who can't afford the training their dogs need. Or sometimes one method doesn't work for a certain dog. Whatever the case is, we want to be able to help people and dogs the way they really need it, versus just making a sale.

So when Pets Strong approached us, it was a no-brainer. We didn't have to run it by anyone; we just went for it. We have fully integrated CBD into our assessment and training program. First, we start out with a free evaluation at the client's home. We determine how severe any possible aggression or anxiousness is and what the best route for training and treatment will be.

One of our first questions to the client--especially if they have an older dog--is: "is your dog healthy? Have you taken them to the vet to rule out any pain or other physical issues?" We also make sure they are in the proper condition to handle the brainwork required for training."

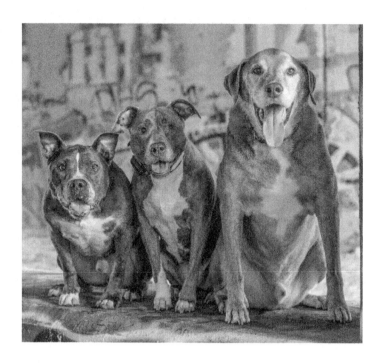

"If they aren't 100% physically, we have to modify or re-consider training. This also could be an indicator of CBD possibly being useful to manage pain.

In one instance, we had a dog named Ziggy in our board and train program who was super anxious--almost borderline aggressive because of his anxiety. I called his owner and got approval to try the CBD on him. And within the first two days, he was coming out of his shell more, he was being more responsive to people approaching him, and was better about getting in and out of the kennel. It ended up being a total turnaround for him because he really opened up and took to the training a lot better. He was more relaxed overall and wasn't so worried about what was going on around him, so to speak. His owner kept him on it after the program, too, so he still gets it every day and is doing well.

And then there was another dog named Remington who was truly aggressive, and they've been using the CBD as well, and it's definitely done good things for him. He's calmed down and relaxed, and is not so responsive or reactive.

Then, aside from our business, everyone in our uses it! Matt, all of our kids, and I take it every day!

Matt and I use it mostly for inflammation, better sleep, and pain. When you wrestle dogs all day long, at the end of the day, you're feeling pretty rough. On top of that, I was a groomer for six years, so I have old back, wrist, and knee injuries.

I not only use the oil, but I also use the cream as well. It's amazing on my wrists. When the weather starts to kick up is when I really start slathering it on.

And it's helped with my migraines. Instead of popping a bunch of over-the-counter meds, I usually will just take a dropper of the oil and rub some of the cream on my neck, and probably within 20 minutes, I'm a new person.

As for my kids, my oldest has ADHD, and it really helps him to focus during school time. And my middle one is the one with autism. It helps him process things more easily. On days he's acting a little extra wild in class, his teacher will text and ask me if I forgot to give him his oil, and then I'll run over to the school and give it to him.

And she'll notice within probably about an hour, he just slows down--evens out, almost. It stops letting his brain go wild, and he's actually able to focus a lot better.

My youngest Freya is almost two, and she gets in line at night before bed, and she just opens her little mouth and says, "Ahh." And I squirt some in there, and it helps her sleep like a champion.

I love that PetStrong's formulas for humans and pets are the same, besides the peppermint being added to the people version. It's funny, though--my oldest and middle kids don't like the peppermint, so I actually give them the dog version because it doesn't have any flavor to it.

It's helped everybody in my family and our clients. It's priceless. So we are big fans and advocates. I think everyone can find use for it, but I do have to say: do your research. It absolutely matters where it comes from; Amazon does not have the good stuff."

For more information about Candice dog training
https://www.awedogtraining.com/
https://www.facebook.com/AWE.DogTraining

Chapter Twelve

Seizures
Pet Parent CBD Stories

Ace Finds Relief from Seizures

"I am a Cannabis Advocate. I had a severe spinal injury in 1976 and have used cannabis when needed ever since and avoided debilitating spinal surgery. I am healthy and happy at 69 years of age and have outlived both of my parents. Cannabis cures so many ailments--in both the human and dog world.

I give my own senior dachshunds CBD for several things, including seizures. Ace is 13 and Daisy is 14. Ace began having seizures when he was 6 months old. Daisy is healthy and has never had seizures, but arthritis set in about 3 years ago and I dose her for that. It helps her get around.

During his seizures, Ace used to fall over stiff and have difficulty breathing. He would regain his balance, then he would purge himself of all stomach contents, then urinate and defecate. These episodes would last about 5 minutes. He had no control over it.

Over the years, his vets have prescribed different medications, but nothing ever worked on him. He battled his seizures all his life, up until about 3 years ago. I found some CBD oil specifically made for pets at a clinic, and that changed everything.

Because I come from an era when a jail sentence resulted from possession of cannabis, I was afraid at first about using CBD on the dogs. I was afraid I would be found out and charged with cruelty to animals. "

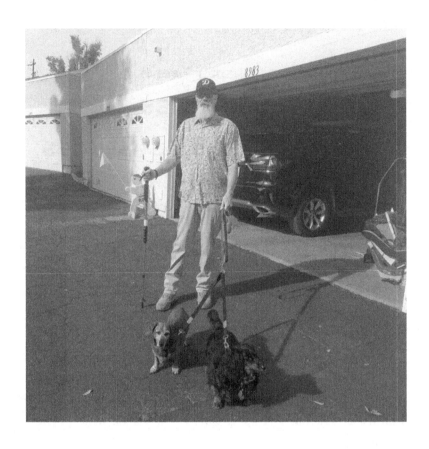

"Now as we know, that would be a total misunderstanding of this amazing herb, but it (and worse) has happened to people. So I was nervous the first time I tried it, but the thing is, dogs have a way of showing and teaching us about the value of unconditional love. If I ever need a true friend, I go to my dogs. They are always there for me, and I had to do this for them.

Within a few days of starting the CBD, Ace's seizures ceased. He's responded well to it; he has experienced no negative effects, and the same is true for Daisy. Getting them to take it has never been an issue--I either put it directly into their mouths with a dropper, or give it to them on some of their kibble, and they take it with no problems.

Ace is doing really great for his age. He's a happy little guy who loves his walks. Daisy too. They just love to walk and we do that without fail, rain or shine. My primary concern was always Ace's well-being and since he has no more seizures when I give him his CBD one time a week as maintenance, I am happy for him. It fills me with joy that he his free of his debilitation.

The one piece of advice I would share is: the cost for CBD oil (particularly if it has THC in it) can be quite high. If you can find a vet that will advise you, and is able to help you find a product that is affordable, go that route.

Otherwise (and I'm sure this advice can't actually be endorsed by any company, but I'm speaking for myself, so I'm just going to say it), I say make your own and save $80 plus. There are instructions online."

Harley Fight With Seizures is Helped With CBD

I adopted Harley, a 9-year-old terrier mix, from my friend when he was 9 weeks old. About 18 months ago, Harley was diagnosed with epilepsy (seizure disorder). The vets prescribed phenobarbital for him, but after reading about all of the side effects it had, I researched other alternatives.

I did pick up the medication from the vet, but I never gave it to Harley. Instead, I visited a local dispensary and had a long talk with the owner, who told me all about CBD, and even shared her experience with using it for her own seizures.

I told her I was scared to try it because I didn't want to make him feel "high" or drugged up, and I was so worried I would overdose him. But she assured me it was nearly impossible to do that. I was sold! I bought a bottle and began experimenting to find the right dose.

I started with too high of a dose at first--Harley was really lethargic-- so I decreased it, and found the sweet spot that helped reduce his seizures, but didn't make him extra sleepy. He gets 5 drops, twice a day in some yummy cooked chicken that he gobbles down easily.

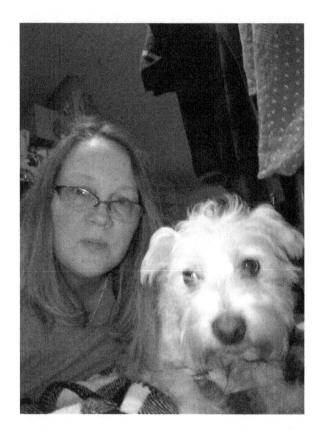

At first, my vets were not very open to her treating Harley with CBD, but I have stuck to it, and I keep a log of what dosages he receives and when, and when he has seizures. They seem to be coming around: they have commended me on helping Harley and staying on top of the situation. I think more and more vets are realizing there are alternative ways out there!

Harley went from having 4-5 seizures a week before the CBD to 1-2 a week after starting it. Then they went down to 2-3 per month. Knock on wood, it has now been 6 weeks since his last seizure!

It is very stressful on both of us when he has a seizure. He knows when it is coming on and will alert me so I can help him through it. I pick him up and lay him on my bed and just hold him tight to let him know that I am there with him. I talk to him and let him know he will be ok. Those moments are getting fewer and far between though, because

Harley is now doing great, thanks to the CBD. He is a happy-go-lucky, friendly dog. He is my little shadow; he likes to be wherever I am. That said, now that we are having such great success with CBD, I don't worry so much about leaving him during the day while I work.

Chapter Thirteen

Get Old without the Aches
Pet Parent CBD Stories

Antonio Finds His Joy Again

Antonio is my heart and soul. He's a 12-year-old rescue Italian Greyhound, and he's my service dog. It didn't start out that way; it just kind of happened. Several years ago, I noticed that he would go into a kind of "guarding mode" where he would randomly put his back to me and sit down and not let anyone else near me. Then I would collapse shortly thereafter.

I live with many diseases, and I have trouble regulating my body temperature, which is what causes the fainting spells. Once I started "listening" to Antonio's cues, I could get myself into a safe spot.

Once I went on permanent disability, I worked with him to hone these skills so we can be out in public, and he has saved me time and time again. He does other tasks, but this is the most important and life-changing one.

When he was 2, he broke his leg and had to get a plate put in. It's been great, but that was 10 years ago. About 6 years ago, he started limping on it. I took him to the vet to see what they could do, but all they told me was *"yes, it is probably arthritis."* They didn't offer any help beyond that.

In 2017, I learned about CBD when I was researching solutions for my own anxiety. It actually didn't help me, unfortunately, but I tried giving it to my four dogs (including Antonio) when I saw all of my friends giving CBD to their dogs for anxiety.

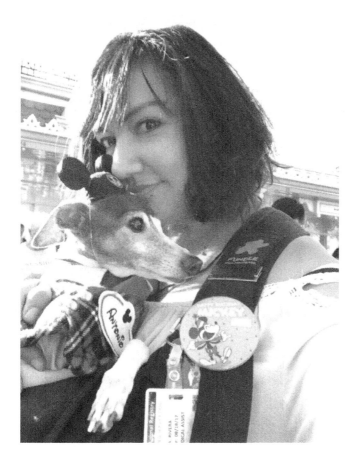

Literally within a couple of days of starting the CBD, Antonio had completely stopped limping, even when he was naked and it was freezing in the morning (which is when he limped the most). I was truly amazed! I accidentally skipped ONE DAY and the very next day, he was limping again. It breaks my heart to see him this way, so I will always make sure I don't accidentally skip a dose. Also, my other dogs are less anxious when I leave them at my mom's house to babysit. It's really a win-win. He also has had a few seizures in his past. I'm hoping that with the CBD, they are totally gone for good.

I love Antonio's spirit. He loves to play...which he wouldn't do much when he was in pain. Now he has that freedom again. I love to take him on walks in beautiful areas...parks, gardens.

I love to play catch with him, too. I feel so much less stressed about Antonio. I always worried I wasn't doing right by him. Always worried he was in pain. Now I'm more at ease knowing I finally found something to help. When CBD didn't work for me...and when the dogs wouldn't touch that first oil...I had my doubts about all the hype. Now I see proof right in front of me that it works. I am truly a believer!

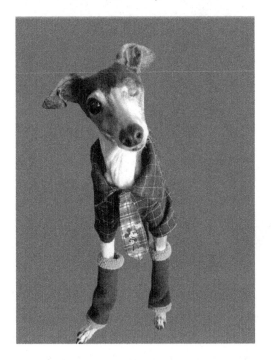

Clove Finds Relief From Motion And Fluidity Problems

"My dog Clove is part German Shepherd, part Boxer. She was a rescue pup. I rescued her when she was three-months-old. She's a handicapped dog with a bowed front foot and incomplete muscle and tissue in-between her two front legs. She had so many problems with motion and fluidity resulting in pain for her.

She'll be eight-years-old next month. I've tried everything I could think of. I've tried baby aspirin. Some very expensive glucosamine cookies from the vet. Nothing made a difference. I tried the CBD oil with a completely open mind. Within two to three days, saw an improvement, and have continued to see an improvement every single day since then.

The fluidity in her motion is much better. Her creaky noise that used to just make me insane is gone. I haven't heard it at all. Now, she's just a happier dog. She likes it. I put it in her food at dinner time, and she enjoys it. She waits for it, she waits for the dropper to come out and knows I'm going to put that in her food. And just her overall health has vastly improved. She's so much more relaxed and she's so much happier, and I don't see any physical pain in her at all."

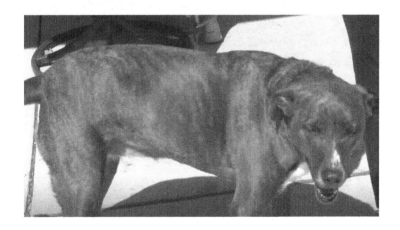

Rocky Ages without Pain

My dog Rocky is a Miniature Pinscher, just over 15 year old. For the past couple of years we have noticed he is starting to slow down, as they will. In the mornings, he does not want to go outside to go to the bathroom. More and more he will just want to lay in his kennel more often. If we did let him out of his kennel, he'd just pick a corner in the house and stay there. We have other dogs, and he just wouldn't want to participate with them and also coughing a lot.

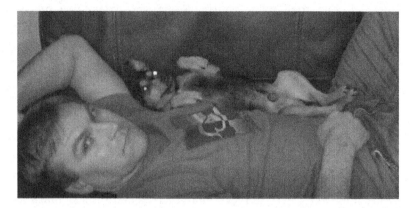

I don't know what the reasoning is, but he'd cough quite a bit. We decided to try some CBD Oil to see if it would alleviate some of his symptoms and to my surprise, it worked effectively and quickly.

Within about the first week and a half, we started noticing the coughing was gone, and in the mornings he gets up out of his kennel and runs to the door. And it seems like he's not in as much pain. I'm assuming he's probably got arthritis. And he's a lot more active and just more happy-go-lucky. Taking away the pain is the main reason why he's so much more active. So hopefully we'll be able to get quite a few more years, hopefully.

Finding Relief from Back Injury Pain

"My pet is a Maltzu, a Maltese Shih Tzu, a very small, 10-pound dog and he hurt his back. For five or six years now, he has problems with his hind legs and motion. Before CBD, I took him to the vets and I left pretty discouraged because they had nothing for him for his pain other than pain medication which I didn't want to give him.

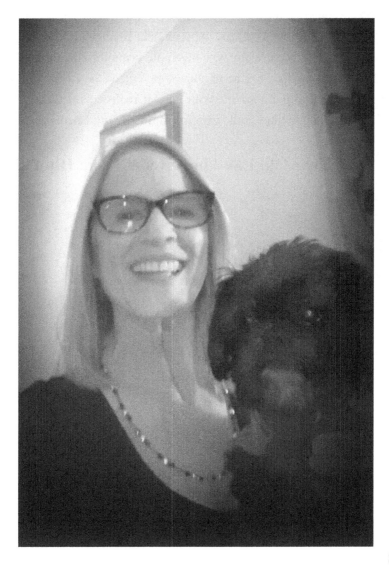

S
o I tried the CBD Oil and he was able to jump back up on the couch, up and down the stairs, running and playing like he always had, and this happened within the first week of me giving him this oil. So I've been giving it to him ever since. The oil is keeping him flying up and down the stairs, he can even run now whereas, he could barely walk.

Before he was hurting to the point where he was almost dragging his hind legs. Now he's walking; he's running; he's doing everything, not as quickly of course, but he's doing everything that he used to do, so I'm so happy. There's no need for any type of pain medication for him at all anymore. I don't even use any type of supplements for him anymore.

I had him on like a glucosamine supplement, he doesn't even use that. It's been a miracle for me with him. It really has. I would highly, any age dog, I do believe could benefit from CBD oil. I really do."

14 Year Old Lab Finds Relief From Hip Pain

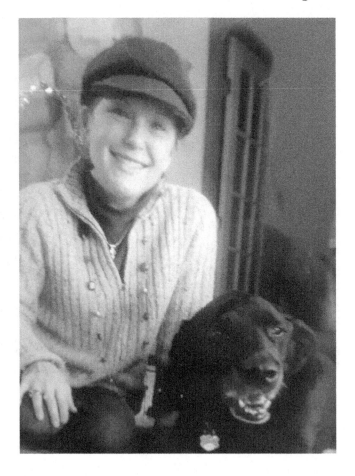

"Kobe is my 14-year-old black Lab, and he, just with age and breed, was having real issues with his hips, and wanting to but having a hard time in getting up and moving around. We took him to the vet and they want to put him on this drug, that drug, or worse telling me that he's just old and euthanize him for his betterment. And I didn't believe that that is necessary.

So I got some CBD oil about two months ago to try out. Started out and now he is a new dog. You wouldn't even know he's 14. Every morning he gets up and greets me. Whereas before around Christmas time, he wouldn't even wake up, I'd have to go wake him up and get him moving. Now he's getting right up, coming out, greeting me just like he used to last year.

It has been a nightmare taking him to the vet again and again. Just the expenditures to see the vet are in the hundreds, walk in the door, before you even get anything. And then their regimen of special dog food or this or that, which even though I see it help animals but minimally. Not enough to warrant all of that expenditure.

After trying CBD for last couple of months, my expenditure in comparison is tenth... Not even half as much. And for the results, it's priceless. I would pay a lot more than what I would to see my dog and have him back.

And also, I used to have to put earplugs at night to sleep (they are both snoring in my ears) in between the dog and my husband. And now I only have to wear them in one ear because the dog is on this side and my husband's on this side, the dog is not snoring anymore and my husband is still snoring. LOL."

Mrs. Beasley and Walter Fight Off Soreness & Accident Pain with CBD

"Mrs. Beasley, a teacup mastiff, my other dog, (Yes I know I have strange names for my dogs.) So she over-exerted herself playing out in the yard and she came in limping and that progressed and she was really sore and she was laying down and I couldn't really get her to get up and I was really scared that she had might have torn her ACL. She's very athletic and only 150 pounds.

And I gave her some of the CBD oil for the next few days. She was getting a little bit better, a little bit better, and it was almost about four days that she was on it, and it was a Saturday, and I said, to my husband, I said, "Okay, if she is not marked better by tomorrow, I'm going to take her into the vet, x-ray, see what's going on." Because in my experience and in my past I'm the first to run to the vet, and I get a $500 bill, and then the next day the dog is fine. And I'm like, "Really?"

Mrs. Beasley

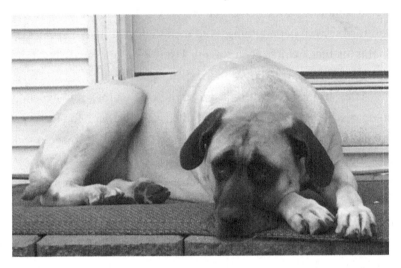

So I put her on CBD and I was hopeful but not expecting because she was sore. I mean she was really miserable. And then sure enough, so that was Saturday, I said, "Okay." And Sunday would be day five. And sure as heck did she just get up and start walking around. I'm like, "Are you kidding me?" And I'm just thankful that I waited and used CBD, and I was rewarded with it and she was rewarded with it, and she's fine. Now it's been since last week and she's fine, running around outside, wouldn't even know that she just got injured."

"My other dog, I have an American Mastiff, his name is Walter and he is 3 1/2 years old, is in great health. Unfortunately, one night he chased a deer out into a road and got hit at about 15 miles per hour, by a car, which dragged him, and rolled him, and we raced him to the vet and they did X-rays. There was no problems, lot of swelling, lot of abrasions but we were very fortunate.

And it's because he's 240 pounds of monster puppy. And things seemed fine but as... I started to notice that when he was laying down as time progressed, he'd start growling, and crying and I brought him back to the vet, asked him to do another set of X-rays, they couldn't find anything and they cleared all of his X-rays. And so, I realized that he had some kind of damage that couldn't be seen, couldn't be felt, it couldn't be replicated unless he was laying down, and even then.

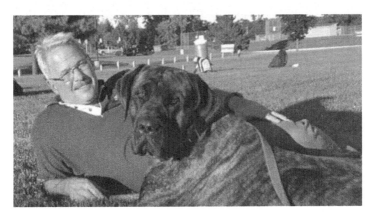

So, we put him on some stronger medicines. I was not really thrilled with that prospect. It causes some side effects, kidney side effects that can happen. And he was too young for me to start him on that regime, I felt. And when this CBD came along, I felt that was a really great option for him.

I've had other friends who feel that they've had success with CBD but I've been very cautious. A lot of places you don't know where it comes from, you don't know whether it's organic, if it's truly organic, but with Pets Strong CBD I felt confident that I knew where it came from.

And I felt that I trusted the source it came from, so that was a good option for me to go ahead and start administrating it to Walter.

So, he has been on it. In the beginning, when he lays down is when he always has symptoms. It's when the growling comes, there could be no one around him and he will growl on himself. He'll get up and go towards his back legs and he's not had that at all.

That was such a huge relief to me. And it made me an absolute believer that there is something to be said about something that's organic, and it's holistic and it's not made in a pharmacy, but made in nature that really has given a second lease on life. And that makes me happy. Dogs are happy, I'm happy. When I'm happy, my husband's happy. If I'm not happy, my husband's not happy. Dog's not happy, then I'm not happy, then the husband's definitely not happy. So, it's a win-win. It's kind of like marriage therapy in a little bottle with drops you give your dog."

Popeye finds his Spinach (in CBD)

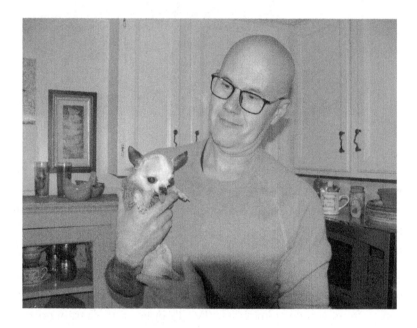

"Popeye, my dog, he is an 11-year-old Teacup Chihuahua. And for the past several years, just from being older, he's had a lot of arthritis problems. And for a couple of years, he's been constantly licking his paws. And trying to solve that issue with food, and some other supplements didn't quite work. But we gave him the CBD and after a couple of weeks, he stopped doing it, to such an extent, that all his hair has grown back on his paws. He had pretty much licked it all off.

Also, he was a lot more lethargic, because I think he was in pain. And so any time he needed to get into his bed because he has a ramp going up to his bed, and also there are stairs in one of the rooms, and so he can't get from one part of the house to the other without going up the step, and he refused to do it.

He'd just sit there and bark, and we had to go and pick him up, so we were basically moving him around everywhere because he just didn't want to walk. And now he has a lot more energy, he acts more like a little puppy than he has in a long time. And he just seems much more comfortable.

Before we gave him the CBD oil, it was a hit or miss if he wanted to eat or not, because some dogs are a little bit more fussier than others, but lately he just really didn't want to eat anything, he might've been in pain, maybe they had upset his stomach.

He would throw up sometimes before he even ate. And you would think, "Well, he's hungry then," but I think he was in just so much turmoil from being in pain, from your arthritis and all that, that he just wasn't hungry, it upset his stomach. So after we gave him the CBD oil, he was on it for a while, for a couple of weeks, his appetite came back. He's not really fussy, anymore. He's just a lot more content, a lot more laid-back.

And another thing is, he has an issue with sound, loud sounds like rain and thunder, he gets terrified. Some dogs get completely terrified, there's nothing you can do, that's horrible. If it's raining at night he'll just start barking and pacing and that'll keep my wife and I up all night too, it was terrible. So we would always dread when it would be raining outside.

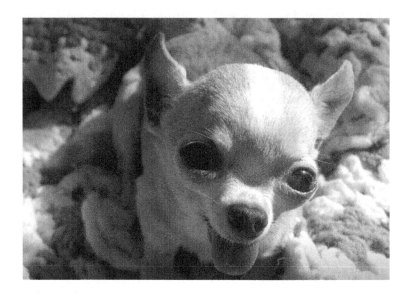

And we noticed that since he's been on the CBD, he doesn't have that problem anymore. It could be raining outside, it could be rain against the windows, thunder, he just sleeps right through it. It's really amazing."

Dexter and Bladder Issues

This past July, my cat Dexter started suffering from anxiety-induced bladder issues that made it difficult for him to urinate. He was peeing blood and repeatedly attempting to use the litter box, even though not much would come out, so we took Dexter to the vet. They did a series of tests that came back negative for cystitis and other infections. T

They sent us home with 3 cans of Royal Canin Urinary SO prescription cat food and a prescription for Gabapentin, which did not seem to be effective. The cat food may have helped, although I was suspicious of the processed ingredients since Dexter has been on a raw meat diet his whole life.

By then, it had been a week, and we were looking for some other options. We consulted our holistic vet (Dr. Rachael Feigenbaum at Lotus Vet in San Francisco), who suggested that Dexter's bladder problems were an issue commonly experienced by anxious or stressed-out felines, and that this issue that can often be resolved with CBD. I was totally on board to try it for Dexter since I use it myself!

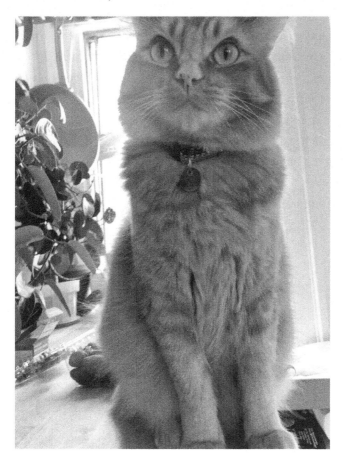

It was hard to get him to take the oil at first, but once I got it in him, Dexter made immediate improvement. Within two days of starting the CBD, Dexter stopped peeing blood, and within 3 days, he was no longer struggling to urinate. He also seems less anxious or stressed out. Now he doesn't mind taking it, and kind of seems to like it! We use a very high quality brand only available in California that has a 30:1 ratio. We give it to him once a day in the morning by putting 4-5 drops on a finger and rubbing it in his cheek for about 30 seconds. I understand this is a more effective method than eating CBD, due to different absorption rates.

Since putting Dexter on CBD, aside from no more bladder issues, he's noticeably less high-strung, less jumpy, and will tolerate being held for longer amounts of time. Plus, it's awesome to see Dex playing fetch with his fuzzy mice again.

A funny thing is, Dex has started kind of liking medicine time, so it's possible he associates CBD with feeling better (although it's hard to know for sure). Since he takes to it so well, we may keep him on CBD for the rest of his life. A couple of drops of CBD per day is very cheap, so cost is not an issue.

Dex is such a loving, attentive boy, and his quality of life has improved so much. He's a much more relaxed and easy-going kitty, which makes me happy! I want this him and his big ginger coat of floof to be around and healthy for a long time!

Chapter Fourteen

How Cannabinoids Can Help Dogs Live a Healthier Life
by Adrienne Wisok

"I have known about CBD for a while now, and have actually studied it in depth. I'm a dog trainer and largely work with sporting and working dogs, and dogs who have very serious behavior problems and work on helping them feel better and less afraid.

I hold a master's degree in service dog training, but before I became a full-time trainer, I worked as a vet tech for 20 years and started a PhD in Neuroscience at UCLA. We studied the use of cannabinoids as a way to relive chronic pain relief that didn't negatively affect the central nervous system, like opioids do.

Cannabinoids are just about everything that we associate with the cannabis plant. This includes CBD, THC, and all of the other molecules in the plant. It turns out that there are receptors for those molecules on every cell in our human bodies, which makes them a really great subject for a lot of different kinds of research.

Through our study, we found that although opioids are great for short-term treatment, they are a really poor choice for long-term pain management. One of the reasons is your body gets used to them and they become less effective over time. This is called physiologic tolerance.

As part of that physiologic tolerance, the receptors in your body for opioids are actually down-regulated in chronic states of pain, which means you have fewer and fewer receptors available to even access for those opioids to be effective at all.

Unlike opioids, cannabinoid receptors are upregulated in states of chronic pain. So not only do you not have the same physiologic tolerance because it's not an addictive substance, you also have more and more receptors, so cannabinoids become more effective over time for chronic pain relief than any other medication. It's the only thing that we know that does that.

In terms of cats and dogs, they have very similar physiology to us. The only real difference that we have to think about when it comes to using CBD on them is that they are smaller than us, so we have to dose by their body weight.

Of my two cats and three dogs, I currently just have my three-year old German Shepherd Taff on CBD. We've had him since he was one, and he's always had a ton of anxiety. He is really, really glued to me all the time. I've tried about four different medications on him, and they either didn't work, or the side effects were too great.

Some of these meds don't get rid of the anxiety at all; they just sedate him so much that he doesn't really move around. Acepromazine was like that. It didn't make him less anxious, so he would still whine, but just get really sleepy at the same time.

I started him on CBD when he was about a year-and-a-half old. It hasn't transformed him into a totally normal dog, but he doesn't seem to want to jump out of his own skin anymore. It hasn't changed his personality, but he's calmed down and seems a little more okay with what's going on in the world instead of being constantly vigilant and worried about everything.

I found Pet Strong because of a dog training facility that I used to work with. The owner was using Pet Strong for her dog who was extremely reactive and sensitive. He was terrified out on walks, he was terrified of dogs, he was terrified of people.

CBD changed her life with her dog. She can now take him out for long neighborhood walks again. His reactivity has not gone away, but he's able to tolerate a lot more. He's still the same dog, but he doesn't have those panicky moments where he's terrified of the world. And she started taking the Pet Strong for humans and said it was hugely helpful for her anxiety and her chronic pain.

I also volunteer for Bark Nation, an all-volunteer non-profit organization that houses dogs who are what we call live-evidence seized from abuse, neglect, or dog fighting. We rehab them and adopt them out when they are ready.

There are so many applications for CBD and it's so much safer than the alternatives, I feel like people would be remiss to not try it before going with a medication.

Unfortunately, the way our legal system is right now, most veterinarians are not allowed to bring up CBD, which means that the onus is on the individual to really ask about it and learn about it as an alternative modality for what they otherwise might have used pharmaceuticals for.

Meds can take a big toll on pets' bodies. We only have a limited amount of time with these little friends. CBD is so easy and can help so much, we sort of owe it to them to try it.

CBD doesn't harm the liver like a lot of medications do. Typically, pet owners rely on blood tests to warn them of any organ damage. The scary part is that they have to do damage to 60% of their liver before a change will show up on blood work.

So by the time you see that change in blood work, they've already largely destroyed the capacity of their liver. Same thing is true for your kidneys. By the time you know about it, it's almost too late.

Anytime you're thinking of a pain medication or any other psychoactive medication, definitely consider CBD instead or as a supplement. Talk to your veterinarian, and let them know that you're going to try it, and ask dog trainers and veterinary technicians about CBD. Definitely look for a brand like Pets Strong, that actually tests for how much CBD is in there, and uses high quality ingredients.

Even if your pet doesn't have a specific condition, you may want to try it anyway as a wellness practice, especially once they reach middle age, which could be anywhere in the four to eight year range. Over time, you don't always notice the things that your dog isn't doing that they used to do. As a vet tech, I often tell people that when they start noticing their dogs are unable or uninterested in doing some of those things, it's time to think about whether there's something going on with them physiologically. Of course, dogs change in their tastes over time, just like we do, but maybe there's also a component of discomfort.

And we don't really see that until we offer the relief. And then it's like, "oh my gosh, my dog is like a puppy again!" and you realize all the things that they weren't doing before.

Adrienne Wisok MS CVT CPDT-KA
Owner, Animal Intuition Dog Training https://pooch.life/
Education Manager, National Search Dog Alliance
https://www.n-sda.org/
Email: adrienne@monkey.org
To volunteer donate to Bark Nation: https://barknation.org/

Chapter Fifteen

CBD for Pet Parents
by Dr. Adam Fasick, DC

I am a chiropractor in Brighton, Michigan. In my practice, we've used CBD on approximately 25 patients over the last four months to treat everything from anxiety, to sleep disturbances, to joint pain, to diabetic blood sugar regulation, and we even tried it on a patient that was 83 years old, for Parkinson's tremors. Unfortunately, out of all those patients, only the Parkinson's patient did not get the result he was looking for, but he did get better sleep. Everyone else is having tremendous results. CBD is giving these patients an increased quality of life.

I have patients with rheumatoid arthritis who had been taking Advil & Motrin every day for their pain. They started using CBD oil instead, and it immediately improved their pain levels and decreased the stress on their liver and stomach. Unlike Ibuprofen and Motrin, there are no known side effects of the CBD oil so it's a much more natural alternative.

Lisa is a 50-year-old female suffering from rheumatoid arthritis. She's had rheumatoid arthritis for 20 years, she's been on Methotrexate, Motrin, Ibuprofen, Tylenol--anything she can to fight that pain. I put her on CBD oil, and it has helped her reduce her intake of Methotrexate, helped her get off of the Motrin and the Tylenol on a daily basis, and it's a more natural standard form that her body receives better. She doesn't have side effects to worry about.

In addition to the traditional tincture oil, CBD also comes in a topical cream form. I find that my patients who use the cream--whether it be for arthritis or muscle pain--get immediate relief, typically within 20 minutes of application. Some people use both the oil and the cream. The tincture oil helps with overall inflammation, whereas the cream provides site-specific immediate relief.

I applied the cream to a patient's knee during an appointment and then we chatted for a few minutes. He suddenly asked, "Is it possible my knee pain could be gone already?" I said, "Absolutely", and it was gone, just like that.

I have patients who use it on sore muscles in their back after an active weekend. They come in, use the cream, they get their adjustment, and off they go, feeling better. In my practice, I often use the cream in conjunction with pulse electro-magnetic therapy. Since that penetrates impulses ions into those damaged cells, I've found it gets the cream into those cells more quickly and it lasts longer than just applying it topically.

I also personally use both the tincture and cream for my shoulder pain. In 2009, I was in a car accident and had to undergo shoulder surgery. To this day, I still have joint pain there. Since using the CBD oil and cream, my joint pain has reduced significantly. There are times I am actually pain-free. I get immediate relief that gets me through my day at work.

Another byproduct we find with CBD oil is better sleep. With an increased amount and quality of sleep, our bodies function much better, we don't have the stress and tension in our joints and muscles, we're refreshed, and we're energized and able to do all the things we want. Whether it's playing golf, visiting with grandkids, traveling, or just enjoying their days without pain, CBD oil helps my patients achieve their health and overall life goals.

But the catch is, not all CBD is created equal. We use Relief Strong CBD oil which is organically farmed in Kentucky, but some people tell me they can get it cheaper online or at the gas station or somewhere. But you have to be careful.

You need to know what you're putting into your body to be healthy. There are a lot of companies that use an ethanol-based solvent to extract the oils out of these plants. Relief Strong, however, uses a CO_2-based extraction method, which means I don't have to worry about any foreign solvents inside my oil. I know I'm getting a pure hemp oil.

You also want to use a full-spectrum oil that contains all the nutrients and vitamins, versus an isolate-based oil, which is condensed down to a powder and then reconstituted with additional oil. There is a time and a place for an isolate-based CBD.

Full spectrum is what you should take orally, and your creams should be isolate-based, as you need a carrier oil or cream that will help your body absorb it.

Testing is very important too, not just at the farm but also third-party supplemental testing to insure that I as a consumer know what's in every bottle of product that I buy and I appreciate that I can give it to my patients in good faith.

If you're using a company that it isn't giving you test results, and giving you access to what's actually in their product, I suggest you stop and find a more transparent company.

Dr. Adam Fasick, DC
https://www.drfasick.com/

Chapter Sixteen

What CBD Type is Best for your Pet?

Hemp and the oils have been around for thousands of years yet new to the world. As pet parents all around the world try to understand hemp's wellness benefits, the hemp industry is working very hard to confuse the heck out of everybody with its ever changing jargon about CBD products.

In this chapter, we are going to teach you how to differentiate between different type of CBD products available and which one in our research is perfect for pets wellness.

Hemp oil; CBD Isolate or Distillate; Broad Spectrum CBD and Full Spectrum CBD are the current types of CBD products that pet parents can buy for their pets and for their use. Lets see what each one of these term means and how they relates to the quality of the CBD interacting with your pet's Endocannabinoid System.

Hemp Seed Oil

Extracted from hemp seeds just like olive oil is extracted from olive seeds, it is a nutrient-rich oil that is typically cold-pressed without any chemical processes. Different cultures around the world have bene extracting hemp seed oil and using it for various purposes for thousands of years just like olive oil or mustard seed oil.

Here is the kicker about the many hundreds of Hemp Seed Oil products claiming to have wellness benefits: Just because a product contains hemp oil, it's not necessarily going to contain CBD. Hemp seed oil contains zero cannabinoids — free of THC and CBD. So next time when you pick up a hemp seed oil product at your local supermarket or find one at Amazon, notice these products typically do not label "dosage." Hemp seed oil is non-psychoactive, non-psychotropic, and non-intoxicating.

Because hemp seed oil is a food product, products containing strictly HSO are federally legal, and have been regulated by the FDA for decades.

So if hemp seed oil contains no CBD, why are consumers buying it and why people have been extracting it over the centuries? Well even though it contains no CBD, when applied topically, hemp seed oil has good properties as a natural moisturizer: deeply hydrating, non-comedogenic (won't clog pores), and is naturally absorbent.

Another use of hemp seed oil: It is often used as a carrier oil (because of its absorbent qualities) in full-spectrum, broad-spectrum, and isolate CBD based products.

CBD Isolate

Jokingly referred around my house as the Microwaved CBD, CBD isolate products are created with a chemical extraction process isolates the CBD molecule from the hemp plant extract. In a white granulare powder form, CBD Isolate contains just the singular CBD molecule. There are not any other cannabinoids, terpenes, flavonoids, or fatty acids naturally present in the product unless they were added separately during the making of that product.

So no entourage effect and with its absence, my firm belief that products made from CBD Isolate lack the wellness efficiency that full-spectrum CBD products will provide to a pet. For people however, cosmetic products or pain creams that only require CBD and CBD only, the Isolate provides a good commercial solution to be mixed easily with different compounds that absorb easily through the skin.

Also if a person (fire fighter, pilot, police officer, long distance truck driver) simply cannot even be near THC even in minute quantities yet still want to try CBD for some wellness benefit for themselves – CBD Isolate based products might be the only type of product they can take as the contain 0.0% THC. For pets, who don't have to worry about random drug testing and should be benefiting from the 'entourage effect' – I recommend skipping CBD Isolate based products altogether.

Broad Spectrum CBD

Entirely devoid of THC, broad-spectrum CBD extracts are made in one of two ways:

- THC is chemically removed from the full spectrum extract, or
- CBD isolate is combined with other cannabinoids, terpenes and flavonoids that also separated chemically from the hemp plant extract in an attempt to mimic the full spectrum effect without THC.

So why go through this hassle and more chemical extraction processes when you can just buy a full spectrum CBD product? Five years ago, with hemp still on the illegal list, the only way a CBD product could be made was from importing CBD Isolate powder from Europe. Consumers were still learning about CBD and nobody even knew what full spectrum CBD was.

As CBD products become more popular and mainstream, more and more customers are asking for full spectrum CBD products yet some of them (people not pets) cannot take full spectrum CBD products because of drug testing by their employers.

Some companies are hoping that by combining both (all cannabinoids minus the THC), broad spectrum CBD products will gain traction with people. It may. The jury is still out. Or drug testing results will become smart enough to distinguish between minute trace amount of THC and not flag them as a marijuana by product which will effectively end the broad spectrum CBD marketing play.

Either way I don't believe that broad spectrum presents any viable wellness for pets. It was built to solve a problem that people face. Not pets.

Full Spectrum CBD

The real deal. "Full-plant" or "whole plant" CBD, think of full spectrum CBD is extracted from a process where the entire hemp plant is used for extraction. Everything in the hemp plant: leaf, stalk, and seeds, are processed to make the full spectrum oil. The final product includes all naturally present cannabinoids, terpenes, flavonoids, and fatty acids.

We believe that full spectrum hemp extracts are what nature intended for us to consume. They come with an all-natural entourage effect built right in.

The entourage effect is the thesis forward by many scientists hat the hundreds of compounds in the cannabis plant work synergistically together to provide a wider range of medicinal benefits vs just consuming CBD by itself. Full-spectrum CBD typically comes from hemp plants and will contain 0.3% or less THC.

For pets, I recommend full spectrum CBD products above all. Why give them microwaved CBD or a product with certain compounds added on artificially when nature has already give these pets an opportunity to get all the benefits of the hemp plant via the full spectrum CBD products? For a pet parent, this choice is simple to make.

RESOURCES

CBD Dosage Guide

In some respects, figuring out how much CBD you should give your pet is more of an art than a science. Because of the lack of studies in the US (hemp just became legal in 2019) we have suggested dosages by weight and severity of the pet's condition. Example: a lower dosage is needed for anxiety than degenerate spine disease when the pet is in severe pain.

NOTE: While most CBD product you purchase will come with its own dosing guidelines, experiences can vary. The ideal CBD dose for the pet usually depends primarily on its weight, but it can also be influenced by other factors, such as its age, and any other health conditions it's dealing with.

Unfortunately, because it is not yet regulated by the FDA, no official dosing guidelines for CBD exist. However, there are best practices and general rules of thumb that can be followed.

How much CBD should I Give My Pet?

When determining your pets ideal CBD dosage, the goal is to find the lowest dose that provides the benefits you need with few or no side effects.

Using the dosage chart below, start with the lowest recommended dose for your pets' weight, and gradually increase from there until you see the desired effects. Once you've found that dose, you can stick with it. Studies show that pets do not develop a tolerance to CBD. The only side effect may be your pet becomes tired if the dosage is too high. Easy fix… just lower the dosage. Also, CBD normally reacts quickly, say within 4 to 5 days you should start seeing some relief. If no relief, increase the dosage until you reach the desired health affect your pet needs.

We are showing you our charts with recommended dosages for cats and dogs. Most reputable companies will give you suggested dosage on their box or bottle for each type of pet: cat or dog.

Shake well before using. Use recommended dosage twice daily at AM/PM. Start with lower dose then increase as needed.

FOR CATS - DOSAGE SUGGESTIONS

Cat Weight	Minimum Dosage	Maximum Dosage
1-5 lbs.	3 drops	5 drops
6-10 lbs.	5 drops	9 drops
11-15 lbs.	.25ml	.25ml plus 5 drops

FOR SMALL DOGS DOSAGE SUGGESTIONS

Small Dog Weight	Minimum Dosage	Maximum Dosage
1-5 lbs.	3 drops	5 drops
6-10 lbs.	5 drops	9 drops
11-15 lbs.	.25ml	.25ml plus 5 drops
16-25 lbs.	.25ml plus 5 drops	.50ml

FOR MEDIUM SIZE DOGS
DOSAGE SUGGESTIONS

Medium Dog Weight	Minimum Dosage	Maximum Dosage
30-40 lbs.	9 drops	0.50 ml
41-50 lbs.	.25ml	.50ml plus 5 drops
51-60 lbs.	.25ml plus 5 drops	.50ml plus 7 drops

FOR LARGE SIZE DOGS
DOSAGE SUGGESTIONS

Shake well before using. Use recommended dosage twice daily at AM/PM. Start with lower dose then increase as needed.

Large Dog Weight	Minimum Dosage	Maximum Dosage
60-70 lbs.	5 drops	0.50 ml
71-80 lbs.	7 drops	.50ml plus 5 drops
81-100 lbs.	.25ml	1.25 ml
100 plus.	1 ml	1.50 ml

Again, these are just general guidelines. Some pets need significantly more, while others need significantly less. For example, if your pet is living with extreme chronic pain, they will likely require a higher dose twice daily than a dog or cat that has a fear of loud noises like fireworks that only needs to be taken occasionally to cope with situational anxiety.

Deciding when to give your pet CBD is as important as the dosage. Do I give it once a day or twice a day or more often? may be a question you ask. The when and how much and how do you administer each dosage will depend on what your treating the animal for. This sounds complicated but it's really not, remember we're giving you guidelines and you can always email me at ask@petsstrong.com for more information and guidance.

Example: If your pet has separation anxiety, you may need to give them one large dose in the morning. If your pet has severe pain, you may choose to split your dose up over the course of the day morning and night. I know of some pet parents that give their pets CBD 3 to 4 times a day for short periods of time to combat chemo. It really comes down to the pet and what we are treating them for, so be patient with yourself as you work out the exact dose for your best friend.

How Do I Administer CBD To My Pet?

There are basically two ways to administer CBD, orally and sublingually.

CBD products taken orally, such as treats or capsules take longer to enter your bloodstream, where it begins to interact with your endocannabinoid system (explained in chapter 2). It must go through your digestive system first (which can take 30 to 90 minutes). Warning: most treats have little or very small amounts of CBD in them requiring you to give multiple treats for them to be effective.

CBD oil administered sublingually has a much faster onset, because it bypasses the digestive system and enters your bloodstream directly under the tongue. Users start to feel effects within 5 to 20 minutes.

Not only does the method of administration affect the onset and duration of effects, but it can also affect the size of the dose you need to take. CBD has very low oral bioavailability, so CBD products ingested orally will lose some amount of the CBD through the digestive system.

However, if you're like me, I go for the easy method and put it on my dog's food and use a slightly higher dosage. Some dogs love the taste, actually beg for it and, you just squirt it into their mouths. For others you need to put it on their food. Cats are a little different story most of the cat parents that I know put in wet food. Example: I only know of a handful that do it sublingually because it's too much work.

Dosage Summary

- Your pets body weight, and other medical conditions determines dosage

- Proper dosage takes a little time but is worth the outcome and, start slow increase as needed

- Your administration method: orally or sublingually depends on your personal and pet's preference

GLOSSARY
Key Terms and Abbreviations

Bioavailability
This term refers to the degree and rate at which a drug is absorbed by the body's circulatory system.

Broad Spectrum CBD
Products labeled "broad spectrum" fall somewhere between full-spectrum and isolate formulations. Because they contain terpenes and other beneficial cannabinoids, broad-spectrum products offer some of the benefits of the entourage effect — without any THC.

For those who can't have or don't want to have any traces of THC in their system, broad-spectrum products can be a better choice than isolates. But they're not as effective as full-spectrum products because they lack the full entourage effect of full spectrum CBD oil products without THC.

Cannabidiol or CBD
One of the 113 naturally occurring cannabinoids found in cannabis plants. It's the second most prevalent active ingredient in cannabis, accounting for up to 40% of the plant's extract. CBD does not produce psychoactive effects i.e. you cannot "get high" with CBD.

Cannabidiol interacts with the endocannabinoid system (ECS), part of the nervous system that's thought to play a regulatory role in all kinds of bodily functions, including mood, sleep, and appetite.

Cannabinoid
Not to be confused with cannabidiol (cannabidiol is a cannabinoid, but not all cannabinoids are cannabidiol), a cannabinoid is one of the many chemical compounds that acts on the endocannabinoid system receptors found throughout the body.

These molecules include the endocannabinoids produced naturally in the body and phytocannabinoids from cannabis. The two most well-known cannabinoids are THC and CBD.

Cannabis l. Sativa
A pre-historic family of plants, farmed for marijuana as well as the industrial hemp used for making CBD products. In addition, hemp fiber, hemp seed oil, and food products are also derived and harvested from different parts of the plant.

COA : Certificate of Analysis

An independent lab report from an accredited laboratory certifying the amount of cannabinoids in a given CBD or THC product. This proof of analysis guarantees quality assurance for both the customers and makers of CBD products.

Learning how to read COA will help you avoid mislabeled, low-quality, or fake products. A reputable company CBD will always provide one for every batch of its products. Many States now require CBD products to come with a QRC code that can direct a customer's smart phone to the company's COA on its website.

CO2 extraction
The carbon-dioxide extraction process uses changes in temperature and pressure to create phase changes in carbon dioxide, gently drawing out the plant's beneficial components. The result is clean, safe oil with a long shelf life.

Delta-9 tetrahydrocannabinol or THC
The primary cannabinoid found in cannabis and the one responsible for its psychoactive effects. It works on endocannabinoid receptors in the brain to release dopamine. Endocannabinoid system

Also known as the ECS, the main function of this mammalian system is to maintain bodily homeostasis, or keeping the body balanced even when the external or internal environment changes.

Scientists believe that cannabis is effective, in part, because the phytocannabinoids it contains mimic our endocannabinoids.

Endocannabinoid receptors are found throughout the entire body, and the system plays a part in many of the body's processes, including appetite, stress, sleep, pain, memory, and immune function.

Entourage Effect
Refers to the scientific theory of many cannabinoids and compound in the cannabis plant interacting together with the human body to produce a stronger effect in totality than any one cannabinoid on its own.

Full-spectrum CBD products combine CBD with other naturally occurring terpenes and cannabinoids (including THC) to be more effective than their isolate counterparts that only have CBD.

Ethanol Extraction
Extraction using cold, high-grade alcohol gently pulls all the active compounds from the cannabis plant's cellulose material, resulting in pure, and full-spectrum hemp oil. Oils extracted using this method are further refined via chromatography to remove all remaining traces of ethanol.

Full Spectrum CBD
The whole hemp plant in a bottle, this is CBD with of all the terpenes, cannabinoids, flavonoids, and fatty acids found in hemp, all of which have therapeutic value of their own work together as the enablers of the entourage effect.

Hemp
A strain of the Cannabis l. Sativa plant often grown for CBD products. By USA Federal Law enacted in Farm Bill 2018, hemp used in CBD products must contain less than .3% THC.

Hemp seed oil
Cold pressed from industrial hemp, hemp seed oil is created by pressing the plant's seeds just as olive oil is extracted from olive

seeds. It has no therapeutic benefits but is often used as a dietary supplement and low-saturated-fat cooking oil.

Industrial hemp
Hemp grown specifically for the industrial uses of its products, including textiles, clothing, biodegradable plastic, food, biofuel, and medicine (including CBD). Hemp and its products are legal in the U.S. under the Farm Bill 2018 as long as they contain less than .3% THC.

Farmers are required to test the hemp crop to insure that they are meeting this federal guideline for 0.3% THC in their hemp crops.

CBD Isolate
A CBD concentrate in white powder form, this is 99% pure CBD and CBD alone. To manufacture an isolate, everything contained in the plant matter is chemically removed — including any traces of THC and other beneficial cannabinoids — until only a powder or crystalline form of CBD is left. Isolate products do not provide any entourage effect to consumers.

Phytocannabinoid
The chemical compounds in cannabis plants that mimic the endocannabinoids naturally produced by the body. CBD and THC are examples of phytocannabinoids, but there are at least 113 different phytocannabinoids so far discovered in the cannabis plant, each producing unique effects in the body.

CBG for example has anti-inflammation properties that might help develop skin care products to help people with acne.

Psychoactive
A property that changes brain function by interacting with the central nervous system and results in altered perception, mood, consciousness, cognition, or behavior. THC is the primary psychoactive component in cannabis plants that can get people high.

Sublingual
Latin for *"under the tongue,"* a method for administering drugs by mouth. It involves placing a substance under the tongue, where it can be readily absorbed into the blood vessels and begin to circulate throughout the body. CBD for both pets and humans is considered most effective when taken sublingually.

Terpenes
The skunk smell associated with cannabis. Terpenes are aromatic oils that lend flavors such as berry, mint, and pine to different cannabis strains. More than 100 different terpenes have been identified so far and every cannabis strain has its own terpene profile.

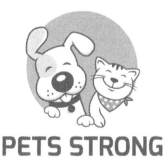

PETS STRONG

CBD From Organically Grown Hemp From Kentucky

Try CBD Risk Free

FREE Shipping | 30 Day Returns

CBD can help your pet with

- ✓ Anxiety (separation, loud noises, fireworks, thunder, travel)
- ✓ Aging Pains (discomfort and aches in joints and bones)
- ✓ Inflammation (itching in skin and coat)
- ✓ Regain Digestion (lost due to chemo or aging)
- ✓ Reduce Reactivity (toward people and other pets)

Made in the USA
Monee, IL
16 January 2020

20410753R00069